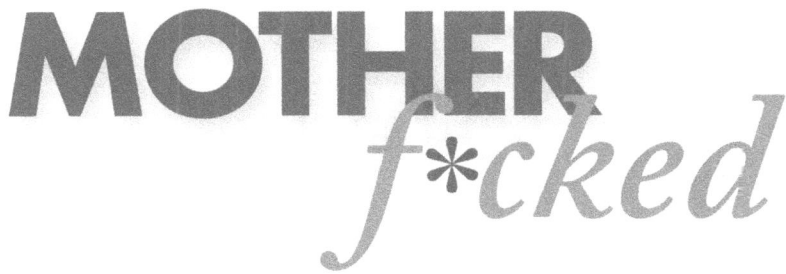

MOTHER f*cked

THE ANTI-PERFECTIONIST'S GUIDE
to Surviving (and Thriving) in the Chaos of Modern Motherhood

REGINA STEELE

ISBN: 9798998960208 (hardback) | 9798998960215 (paperback)

Published by: Mongoose Holdings, LLC
Gilbert, AZ

First Edition
Printed in the United States of America

Disclaimer:
The information presented in this book is for educational purposes only and is not intended as medical advice. The author and publisher shall not be liable for any damages arising from the use or misuse of this material.

Foreword

My daughter, Regina, is one of my best friends. When she told me she was writing this book, I wasn't surprised. I knew it wouldn't be a small undertaking, but it was a deep desire that she had to accomplish. She had done a lot of research and personal practice to reach the place that she is at now. She is my go to person for questions about health and well-being. I am proud of her for reaching out to other moms to help them find their way in a difficult and constantly changing world.

When I was younger, I wish I had known how important it was to set boundaries, use "I feel…" phrases, date my husband, and take time for myself in a busy world. Raising 6 children, doing volunteer work, being a chauffeur, doing laundry, working as a teacher in special education, and taking care of a diabetic child were all part of my day to day. I am sure so many moms can relate.

As Regina's mom, I have seen her work diligently on this book, making it a journey that could lead so many moms to a much happier, and healthier place. Her passion for health, healing, and questioning the system didn't come out of nowhere. In many ways, we've walked parallel journeys. Mine began with a simple conversation at church, where a friend shared how acupuncture had helped her. At the time, I was dealing with chronic back pain, and while I had learned to live with it, I never stopped hoping for something better. That conversation led me to acupuncture, then to chiropractic care, and over time, to an entirely new way of seeing health.

Like so many moms, I was told my pain had only one solution. Shots, prescriptions, and procedures. But I hesitated. Something in me wasn't ready to surrender to that path without exploring others first. I found relief in physical therapy, yoga exercises, acupuncture, and small but meaningful changes in my daily habits. The results were undeniable. My body responded, and I knew I was on the right track. It wasn't always easy, and it wasn't cheap. But, I was determined (and still am determined) to be healthy.

However, my health journey wasn't just about my back. In my 30s, I faced severe depression, hospitalizations, and treatments that often felt like they were managing symptoms rather than healing me. When my son died in 2013, my world shattered. I went through shock therapy, adjusted medications, and fought for clarity when my mind felt like it was slipping away from me. All those "treatments" took a toll on my health in the long run. But, my daughter has always been there to guide me toward the healing path with optimism. She has given me hope when my doctors wanted to make me feel hopeless and doomed. I still see a psychiatrist, but have been maintaining my mental health on 2 medications for several years now.

Healing, I've come to understand, is not one-size-fits-all. It is personal, unpredictable, and often inconvenient. It requires us to listen to ourselves in a world that insists it knows better. This book is a battle cry for mothers who have been told to accept exhaustion as normal, to accept stress as inevitable, and to silence their own instincts. It challenges a system that profits from keeping us just well enough to function, but never truly thrive.

Reading these pages, you will laugh, you will nod along, and maybe, for the first time in a while, you will feel seen. You will also be challenged. Challenged to think differently, to question boldly, and to remember that your health is not a burden or an afterthought.

If there's one thing I hope you take away from this book, it's this: You have more power than you think. Whether it's in how you choose to care for your body, how you advocate for yourself, or how you rewrite the script of what motherhood is supposed to look like—your voice matters. My daughter has written a book that gives that power back to you.

So, take a deep breath, settle in, and get ready. You're about to embark on a journey that just might change everything.

-Toni
(A.K.A. Mom of 6 and Nanni to 10)
Retired Teacher

Introduction

I've always been the kind of person who says yes to adventure. My husband and I live for the challenge: physically, mentally, and in any wild opportunity life throws at us. So when I got pregnant with our first child, I didn't see why I should approach it any differently. I knew from the start that I wanted to go as natural as possible, trusting my body and leaning into holistic methods that made sense. That's when I first dipped my toes into breathwork, body relaxation, and prenatal yoga.

That yoga class? Total game changer. For the first time, I felt deeply connected to the little life growing inside me. Something I never could have expected. My instructor, who was also a doula, became my guide, and with her wisdom, I navigated all three of my pregnancies using yoga as my anchor. Three natural births, no complications, and a feeling of empowerment I wish every mom could experience. I thought I had motherhood and health all figured out.

Then, after my third baby, my body hit a wall.

I was beyond exhausted (like, the kind of tired that no amount of sleep could fix). My energy tanked, my hair was falling out, I dropped weight so fast it scared me, my heart was doing this terrifying fluttering thing, and let's just say my mood was *nonexistent*. I wasn't excited, I wasn't sad, I just felt... nothing. My doctor, in classic fashion, whipped out the prescription pad and suggested a little something for my "depression."

Nope. Not happening.

I had seen too many moms get stuck in the cycle of antidepressants, tweaking doses, adding more meds, and still feeling like shit - just a slightly numbed type of shit. I refused to become another statistic. I needed answers, not a Band-Aid. That's when I turned to naturopathic care, and suddenly, I wasn't just a patient. I was a mom on a mission.

After digging into my health, I discovered the real culprits: Hypothyroidism, Hashimoto's Thyroiditis, Adrenal Dysfunction, and H. Pylori (because why not add a gut infection to the mix?)

With the help of an incredible functional doctor and lifestyle changes that I never learned in a conventional doctor's office, I started to heal. We balanced my adrenals, kicked the H. Pylori to the curb, and stabilized my thyroid—leaving me determined to one day reverse my Hashimoto's entirely. More importantly, I became obsessed with understanding *why* moms are being failed by modern medicine, despite its best intentions.

And that's when I uncovered something even more infuriating: Moms are the least studied demographic in medical research, yet we're the highest marketed to by industries that profit off our exhaustion, insecurities, and struggles.

Big Pharma, the food industry, the beauty industry, even the wellness space; they all have one thing in common: they *sell* to moms while never actually prioritizing our health. They know we make the majority of household purchasing decisions. They know we'll spend money if we believe it will make us better mothers. And they prey on those vulnerabilities. They market toxic skincare under the guise of "self-care," push supplements instead of real solutions, and fill our grocery stores with food that depletes our energy instead of fueling us. They thrive on keeping moms just sick enough, just tired enough, just desperate enough to continue buying their so-called solutions. Solutions that were never designed to actually help us thrive because they are not solutions at all.

And yet, motherhood is the most powerful, life-altering, and sacred position anyone could ever hold.

We are the creators of life. We are the nurturers, the protectors, the healers, the ones who shape the next generation. There is no job, no title, no degree that holds more weight than "Mom." And yet, in a world that should be lifting us up and supporting us, we are instead overworked, underappreciated, and left to figure it all out on our own.

Here's the thing: I *love* being a mom. I love the chaos, the laughter, the deep soul connection that comes with raising tiny humans. And I refuse to accept that motherhood has to be a constant state of depletion. I believe with every fiber of my being that moms can be vibrant, energetic, and strong. We don't have to settle for survival mode.

That's why I wrote this book.

Because I know firsthand what it feels like to lose yourself. To feel like your body has betrayed you and you're trapped in a never ending cycle of exhaustion, anxiety, and overwhelm. But I also know that healing is possible. Not through pharmaceuticals, not through another crash diet or "quick fix," but through knowledge, empowerment, and small, sustainable lifestyle changes that actually work.

Moms deserve better.

This book is my love letter to you, a reminder that you are not broken, you are not alone, and you are absolutely worthy of feeling *well*, not just for your kids, but for *you*. Because when moms thrive, families thrive. And when families thrive, the world changes.

So take a deep breath, grab a cup of something warm (or a glass of something strong), and let's shake off the nonsense we've been sold. You're not just meant to *survive* motherhood. You're meant to *own* it, *love* it, and feel damn good doing it.

With love and imperfection
Regina

"*Mother Fcked** is a breath of fresh air in the media of motherhood. Regina brings a practical, witty perspective on how to retake control of your well-being after becoming a mom. She captures the struggles and joys of motherhood with simple, relatable stories and examples and presents facts about health and nutrition in a captivating and entertaining manner. Her focus on making small changes that have great impact creates an atmosphere of success for anyone inspired to begin the protocol that will change her life. This book will be the motivation and inspiration you need to begin taking those steps toward the healthiest version of you so that you can be more present in every moment of your life.*"
Rosemary, Mom of 2, Ayurvedic Consultant & Yoga Teacher

"*In this book we find truth in the journey of motherhood. The importance of prioritizing self-advocacy for both yourself and your children. Embracing the importance of nourishing your body and mind, ensuring that you can be the best version of yourself for yourself and family. Finding your tribe—like-minded individuals who support and uplift you—creating a sense of community and belonging, and most certainly helping you through the greatest journey, motherhood. And remember that rest is not a luxury but a necessity; it rejuvenates your spirit and empowers you to tackle the challenges of motherhood with grace. By focusing on these aspects, you cultivate a balanced and fulfilling motherhood experience.*"
Deanna, Mom of 2, Yoga Teacher, The Secret Ninja, Super power Queen

"*Mother Fcked hits the nail on the head in so many ways. It's raw, real, and refreshingly honest—without any sugar coating. I found myself deeply relating to its message while also learning along the way. As a firm believer in integrative medicine, I know firsthand that fueling your body with the purest foods can truly be life-changing, and this book reinforces that in the most powerful way.*"
Renee, Mom of 2, Owner of Free and Simple Foods

"*FINALLY someone took my thoughts around food, health, HORMONES; ALL OF IT and put it into a book that I can understand. This book is written in Mom-a-logy which speaks to my mom's heart.*"
Pilar Varela, Mom of Autistic twin teenage boys, Wonder ♀ Woman

"*We all know motherhood is not easy, but damn, does it have to be this hard? This book is a game changer for me. I love the knowledge, humor* *and insight Regina puts into her work. Regina provides great insights with a real and raw take on life, health and how to take control back of your own destiny. We can all thrive and not just feel Mother F*cked."*

Valerie, wife, business owner and mom of 2 collegiate athletes

"Being the nanny of Regina's three children, I have spent quite a bit of time around Regina and her family over the years, experiencing the live action fruits of this book firsthand. When it comes to health, wellness & really anything in the Steele household, Regina comes fully loaded ready to take on the status quo of what is real versus fake in our overly processed, pharmaceutical-obsessed world. Her sharp wit propels her objectives forward, mixed with her ingenuity & no BS attitude—no artificial additives here! She is a force to be reckoned with, and Mother Fcked* embodies every aspect of her badass self & mission to all mothers alike. Just like Regina, this book is a one-of-a-kind and an absolute must read for all the moms out there tired of the same old rat race, same old results. She will change your mindset, and ultimately change your life. I turned the last page feeling a different sense of empowerment with her simple holistic approach that will engage you with pure humor and relatability. If you're ready to take control of your health, well-being and life as a whole, this book will captivate you to do all that—and more!"

Mystique, Nanny of 14 years

"Motherhood is chaos—beautiful, exhausting, and everything in between. As a full-time working mom with three kids running in different directions, I know the struggle of trying to do it all. That's why I'm so excited for my friend Regina Steele's new book, Mother F*cked. Regina gets it— no sugarcoating, no fluff, just real talk, real solutions, and a much-needed reality check on how modern moms are being let down by the system. This book is a must-read for any mom ready to take control of her health, energy, and sanity—without the guilt."

Kate, Mom of 3, Chief Operating Officer at The CSI Companies & also Captain Chaos of the Mays family

"Mother Fcked* felt like a deep breath I didn't know I needed. With honesty, compassion and humor, Regina recounts the messy and beautiful reality of motherhood—leaving me feeling truly seen and understood. As mothers, we all carry a sacred invisible load, but this book brings that load to light. The journey of motherhood is about unwrapping the best version of you and

this book serves as a critical compass to help guide you along the way. Taking care of yourself isn't selfish—it's essential. Prioritizing your health and wellness will allow you to show up more fully for those you love, Mother Fcked* will give you the permission and perspective to do just that."
Danielle, Mom of 3, Chief Memory Maker and Sanity Manager

"Mother fucked is bold, unfiltered and witty! Regina's connection to the cause can be felt in her words, and she paints a spot-on picture of what it's like to be a modern mom. This message made me laugh, cry, and served as a beautiful reminder that motherhood is not meant to be survived; Motherhood is meant to be deeply connected, purposeful and vibrant."
Emily, Mom of 2, Model, Queen of Chaos and Connection

"Regina has taken the time to express her HEART work. This book is for the mom who's exhausted from holding it all together and just wants real answers—not fluff. The one who feels invisible some days but keeps showing up for everyone anyway. I was tired, overwhelmed, and done waiting for someone to help, so I started helping myself. If that's you, too, do yourself a favor and get this book. You deserve it."
Jennifer, Mom of 1

"I have known Regina for many years and I always wondered, "How does she do it?" In "Mother Fcked," Regina lays down the ground rules for how to prioritize not only your family but also yourself. That's right, you CAN do it all. "Mother Fcked" provides the tools for survival, the grace to let go, and the ability to raise a healthy and holistic family in this modern world. Get ready to learn and take charge again! You won't be able to put this book down!"
Candice, Mom of 2

"I enjoyed working with Gina so much and learned a lot about my own health issues! She made me laugh when I wanted to cry and reminded me that I wasn't doing this alone. Gina's words feel like a pep talk, a hug, and a glass of wine all rolled into one. She just gets it—and that's rare and real."
Gianna, Step Mom of 2

"Reading Regina's words feels like taking a deep breath for the first time in a long time. This isn't just a book—it's a lifeline."
Natalie, Mom of 2

"I'm a mom who is endlessly curious about how to support my family's well-being. What I love about Regina and MotherF*cked is how she gets right to what matters—no fads, no fluff, just honest, thoughtful advice that truly helps... and keeps me from spiraling down endless rabbit holes in search of answers. So glad to have her and this book on my side!"

Kelsey, Mom of 2

Table of Contents

Dedication

This book is dedicated to Rick. Thank you for being the most supportive husband and dad. And Ellie, Izzie, and Ethan-Thank you for giving me the most honorable title and position in life:

"Mom"

Part 01

MOTHER *F*cked*

CHAPTER 01

How the F*ck Did We Get Here?

B eing a mom is mental. Am I right?

Mentally taxing. Mentally exhausting. Mentally bruising.

It's 6:00 AM, and before her feet even hit the floor, she's already behind. The baby woke up three times last night, her toddler is demanding the "right" sippy cup (which is, of course, no where to be found), and her inbox is overflowing. Breakfast is a mix of half-eaten toast and spilled milk, all while answering work emails, refereeing sibling fights, and Googling whether that weird rash on her kid's arm is worth a trip to urgent care. By noon, she's powered through deadlines, laundry, and a tantrum over the "wrong" brand of applesauce. By 8:00 PM, she's exhausted but still mentally tallying the 157 things she didn't get done. Rinse and repeat.

Sound familiar?

Being a mom wasn't always this mentally and physically draining. Way back (like *really* way back) being a mother was considered sacred. Moms were respected, nurtured, and supported by their communities. They weren't expected to do it all alone, juggle careers and home life with zero support, or meet impossible societal expectations.

Fast forward to today, and somehow, we've landed in a reality where motherhood is a 24/7 job with no pay, no sick days, and the constant guilt of feeling like we're not doing enough. But why? How did we go from village-supported, honored caregivers to burnt-out, overstimulated, and chronically exhausted martyrs? Let's take a quick look, shall we.

The Loss of the Village. Remember when raising kids was a group project? Yeah, neither do I. Somewhere along the way, the village packed up and left us on our own. In the past, extended families, neighbors, and close-knit communities shared the load. Grandma was next door to help, the neighbor's kid was your built-in babysitter, and everyone looked out for each other's children. Today? Moms are expected to do it all solo, with nothing but a baby monitor and a Wi-Fi signal for support.

This shift isn't just inconvenient, it's unhealthy. The constant demands of child-rearing without communal support lead to burnout, isolation, and mental exhaustion. Depression and anxiety rates among moms have skyrocketed, and yet, we still buy into the lie that asking for help is weakness. The reality? It's how we were meant to function. We weren't designed to parent in isolation, yet society has somehow convinced us that doing everything alone is some sort of badge of honor. Spoiler: It's not.

So, where do we go from here? It starts with rebuilding the village, whether that's leaning on friends, finding community groups, or simply accepting that no, we don't have to do everything ourselves. Because newsflash: humans were never meant to raise kids in a vacuum.

The "Do It All" Expectation. If being a mom came with an actual job description, it would read something like this: "Seeking an individual willing to work 24/7 as a caregiver, chef, maid, chauffeur, financial planner, therapist, tutor, and event coordinator, all while maintaining a thriving career, a spotless house, an Instagram-worthy social life, and a body that 'bounced back' three weeks postpartum." No salary. No benefits. Judgment guaranteed."

Social media only makes it worse. Everywhere you look, there's a perfectly curated version of motherhood that makes real-life parenting feel like failure. The mom influencers somehow manage to make homemade organic lunches, run businesses, and look effortlessly chic. Meanwhile you're just trying to remember if you showered today.

Let's get real: This "do it all" myth is a setup for exhaustion, self-doubt, and chronic stress. The truth? No one is doing it all, at least not without a team of nannies, assistants, and Botox appointments. The key to surviving this madness? Let go of the expectation that you have to be everything to everyone, all the time. It's okay to say no. It's okay to not have a Pinterest-perfect life. And it's *definitely* okay to let the dishes sit in the sink for a night.

Medical Gaslighting. Moms are tired. Like, next-level, running-on-caffeine-and-sheer-will tired. But when we go to the doctor and say, "Hey, I feel like my body is falling apart," we're often met with a condescending smile and a prescription slip.

Exhausted? Must be depression. Here's an antidepressant. Can't lose weight? Eat less, move more. (Wow, thanks, that never occurred to me.) Hormonal imbalance? Just take the pill. Gut issues? Maybe it's in just your head.

Medical gaslighting is real, and it's one of the biggest reasons moms are suffering in silence. Instead of addressing the root causes: nutritional deficiencies, adrenal fatigue, thyroid imbalances, postnatal depletion—many doctors are quick to write off symptoms as stress or anxiety. But here's the thing: of course we're stressed and anxious! We're raising humans with little to no support while navigating a medical system that dismisses our concerns.

Moms need more than temporary solutions. We need doctors who listen, dig deeper, and acknowledge that feeling like garbage *isn't* normal. We deserve better than being handed a prescription and told to "relax".

Toxic Food and Environment. If you look at the average American mom's diet, it's basically a collection of things she can eat one-handed while standing over the sink. And guess what? Most of it is ultra-processed garbage designed to keep us addicted, inflamed, and chronically unwell.

Modern food is a toxic disaster. Between pesticides, preservatives, and artificial everything, our bodies are constantly under attack. And let's not even get started on the environmental toxins. Endocrine disruptors in plastics, heavy metals in baby food, and "fragrance" in every cleaning product (translation: hormone-wrecking chemicals).

Moms are running on empty, and it's no mystery why. Our food, water, air, and daily stressors are all working against us. But here's the good news: we can take back control. It starts with small changes. Swapping out processed junk for real food, choosing non-toxic household products, and understanding that what we put in (and on) our bodies *matters*.

Economic Pressures Have Stretched Moms Thin. Gone are the days when one income was enough to support a family. Now, dual incomes are often *necessary* just to cover the basics. But of course society did not adjust its expectations accordingly. Moms are still expected to run the household like a 1950s housewife while working full-time.

And let's talk about childcare. It's so expensive that many moms are forced into impossible decisions. Keep working and pay a ridiculous percentage of income toward childcare, or quit and lose financial independence. Either way, stress skyrockets, and health suffers.

The Cost of Ignoring This. If we don't take back control of our health, what's at stake? Everything. No, really—everything. We're not just talking about feeling a little run-down or needing an extra coffee to function. Ignoring our well-being has real, long-term consequences, and the price tag is one we cannot afford to pay.

Motherhood has somehow become a survival game, where exhaustion is a badge of honor, and self-care is labeled as selfish. We push through, tell ourselves we'll rest later, and normalize feeling like hell. But "later" doesn't always come, and before we know it, the damage is done.

Let's break down exactly what's on the line when moms put themselves last.

Your Long-Term Health. You know that nagging exhaustion that no amount of sleep (or caffeine) can fix? The brain fog that makes you forget why you walked into a room? The bloating, headaches, irritability, and random aches that seem to be getting worse? Yeah, that's not just *"being a tired mom."* That's your body waving a giant red flag, screaming, "HEY, LADY! PAY ATTENTION TO ME BEFORE IT'S TOO LATE."

Chronic stress, poor diet, and lack of sleep don't just make you tired. They *reprogram* your entire system in ways that lead to serious, lifelong health issues, including:

► **Autoimmune diseases** – Constant stress and inflammation can trigger your immune system to turn against you, leading to conditions like Hashimoto's, rheumatoid arthritis, and chronic fatigue syndrome.

► **Hormonal imbalances** – If your hormones are out of whack, *everything* feels off. PMS becomes a raging beast, metabolism slows, mood swings are next-level, and burnout is just a Tuesday.

► **Metabolic dysfunction** – Blood sugar swings, insulin resistance, and sluggish thyroid function mean weight gain, exhaustion, and that never-ending feeling of *blah*.

▶ **Mental health struggles** – Depression, anxiety, panic attacks, our bodies *literally* cannot regulate emotions properly when they are nutritionally depleted and sleep-deprived.

▶ **Gut health disaster** – The gut is called the "second brain"
for a reason. When it's compromised by processed foods,
stress, and lack of sleep, it throws everything (mood, digestion, immune function) into chaos.

▶ **Increased risk of major diseases** – Diabetes, heart disease,
and even cognitive decline (hello, Alzheimer's) are *directly
linked* to how well we take care of ourselves today.

Basically, if we don't start treating our health like the *foundation* of our lives, it will eventually become the biggest thing
we *don't* have control over.

Ignoring your body's warning signs today can mean spending years down the road fighting to get back what you lost.
And let's be real, *we're too damn busy for that.*

Your Family's Well-Being

Moms are the emotional, mental, and physical *glue* holding
their families together. But what happens when the glue starts
to crack?

Let's not sugarcoat it: when moms are exhausted, overstimulated, and running on empty, the entire family suffers.

▶ **We snap faster** – Your toddler spills a drink, and instead
of calmly cleaning it up, you're ready to scream into the
void. You don't *want* to react that way, but exhaustion and
depletion make it impossible to regulate emotions properly.

- **We're emotionally unavailable** – Your kids want to tell you a story, but all you can think about is how you just need *one minute of peace*. You're present, but not *really* present.

- **We get sick more often** – Burnout weakens the immune system, which means moms are constantly catching every virus their kids bring home. And we all know *moms don't get sick days*.

- **Our relationships suffer** – When we're constantly exhausted, our partners get the worst of us. Conversations turn into complaints, affection takes a backseat, and suddenly, everything feels *harder* than it should be.

- **We model unhealthy habits** – Kids don't do what we *say*, they do what we show them. If we're constantly stressed, skipping meals, neglecting sleep, and never taking time for ourselves, they grow up thinking that's *normal*.

The irony? We pour every ounce of ourselves into making sure our kids are happy and healthy, while slowly sacrificing *our own* health in the process. But if we don't prioritize ourselves, how can we show up fully for them?

Taking care of yourself isn't selfish, it's necessary. Your family deserves the best version of you, not the version running on fumes.

Breaking the Cycle for Future Generations

I'm going to be brutally honest: **the current system is not sustainable**.

Moms today are stuck in an endless loop of exhaustion,

self-sacrifice, and unattainable expectations. And if we don't make changes, both personally and culturally, our daughters will inherit the same **impossible** standards, or worse.

► Do we want them to believe that burnout is normal?

► That motherhood = self-neglect?

► That the only way to be a "good mom" is to give until there's nothing left?

Absolutely *not*.

The best gift we can give our kids (especially our daughters) is showing them what *healthy motherhood* looks like.

► We show them that self-care is non-negotiable.

► We show them that boundaries are a form of self-respect.

► We show them that a mother's worth is not measured by how much she suffers.

By prioritizing our health, we rewrite the story. We raise daughters who know it's okay to rest, okay to ask for help, and okay to put themselves first sometimes. Because when we break the cycle, *we change the future.*

Just because it's normal, doesn't mean it's right
Just because this level of exhaustion, stress, and burnout has become the *default* setting for modern motherhood doesn't mean we have to accept it.

We have a choice.

► We can set boundaries.

► We can demand better healthcare.

- ► We can say no to the "do it all" expectation.

- ► We can prioritize nutrition, sleep, and mental health.

- ► We can call out the societal systems that are failing moms instead of blaming ourselves.

The bottom line? You matter. Your health matters. Your energy, your happiness, your sanity, *they all matter.*

If we don't fight for ourselves, *who will?*

So before we resign ourselves to a lifetime of caffeine-fueled survival mode, let's ask the big questions:

What if we started living motherhood *differently*?

What if we demanded more?

Because the truth is: **we deserve it**.

CHAPTER 02

The Mental Circus of Motherhood

The Mental Load is Real

Balancing multiple roles as a mom is like trying to fold a fitted sheet while blindfolded—with one hand tied behind your back. We juggle careers, parenting, relationships, and household responsibilities, all while society insists we should make it look effortless. The mental battle leaves us feeling like we're constantly running on empty, striving to be a perfect mix of Oprah Winfrey and Betty Crocker.

We're more likely to be low on energy. And things like taking a shower, and eating a full and balanced meal can go out the window. A study with postpartum women found that energy levels for women can stay low for up to **19 months** *(PubMed)* after giving birth. And in my experience, this can last for up to 5 years in many instances-especially after multiple births.

13

Society places an unequal burden on women to be primary caregivers and homemakers, despite professional commitments. This outdated division of labor leaves moms with little time for themselves, leading to burnout and mental exhaustion.

The Science of Mom Burnout

Not that we need studies to tell us what we already feel in our bones, but research actually backs it up: According to the **CDC**, women between 18-44 are nearly **twice as likely** as men to report feeling constantly exhausted. The reason? The relentless physical, emotional, and mental workload of motherhood.

Katie Sardone, Ph.D., a psychologist specializing in burnout, describes it as "a bank account that keeps dwindling. You hit your limit, keep going, and once you overdraft, the fees and fines hit you hard. Moms don't realize they're in the red until it's too late."

Why Society Places These Unrealistic Demands on Moms

So how did we get here? Why do moms carry this enormous burden while society turns a blind eye?

The Perfect Mom Myth – Ah, the Perfect Mom. She's a career powerhouse, a parenting expert, a relationship whisperer, a domestic goddess, and she looks damn good doing it. She packs organic, bento-boxed lunches, maintains a thriving social life, crushes it at work, keeps her house magazine-worthy, and somehow *(somehow)* finds time for weekly self-care. She's got six-pack abs three months postpartum, never forgets a birthday, and has never once locked herself in the bathroom to eat a snack in peace.

And if we're not her? Well, obviously, we're failing.

At least, that's the message society keeps shoving down our throats.

The modern mom is expected to excel in every category. If you're a stay-at-home mom, you should also be running a side hustle. If you're a working mom, you better make every school event, cook from scratch, and never complain about being tired. If your house is a mess, your kids act up, or you choose *yourself* over something "mom-related," get ready for the judgment.

The *Perfect Mom Myth* is a dangerous game, because the reality is, **she doesn't exist**. Not even the influencer moms with their color-coordinated pantries and choreographed morning routines are actually *living* the perfection they portray.

The constant pressure to be more (to be everything to everyone, all at once) has left moms exhausted, anxious, and constantly feeling *less* than. And let's be real: *if* we had the time, energy, and resources to actually try to meet this impossible standard, we'd probably just use it to nap.

It's time to let that fantasy go. *You don't have to do it all to be a good mom.* You just have to be you—messy, imperfect, doing-your-best *you*. And that's more than enough.

The Judgment Culture – Here's a fun fact: **every single parenting decision you make is wrong.**

- ► If you breastfeed, *you're bragging*. If you formula-feed, you're lazy.
- ► If you go back to work, *you're selfish*. If you stay home, you're *unambitious*.

- If you let your kid have screen time, *you're ruining their brain.* If you don't, *you're depriving them of educational opportunities.*

- If you feed them organic, *you're a snob.* If you give them a Happy Meal, *you obviously don't care about their health.*

- If your kid wears mismatched socks to school, *why aren't you paying attention?* If they're too put-together, *why are you so obsessed with appearances?*

Moms cannot win. Every choice is scrutinized, criticized, and turned into an online debate.

And let's not forget the working mom guilt—because of course that comes with an extra layer of judgment. According to a 2022 **Harris Poll**, 42% of working moms are diagnosed with anxiety and depression—a rate significantly higher than child-free women (25%) and even working fathers (35%). Why? Because on top of the crushing weight of doing it all, we're constantly told we're not doing enough.

The result? We second-guess everything. We spiral into guilt. We wonder if we should be doing more, even when we're running on fumes.

Here's the truth: your parenting choices are your own. The people whispering judgments aren't living your life, raising your kids, or carrying your mental load. The only thing that truly matters is what works for you and your family. The judgment culture only has power if we keep buying into it—and frankly, *moms are too damn tired for that.*

Financial Pressures – Let's talk numbers: Raising a child in

2025 costs upwards of $306,000. And that's before you even think about college.

Now add this fun little fact: moms still earn 16% less than men, according to **Forbes**.

So, let's recap:

- ▶ It's more expensive than ever to raise kids.
- ▶ Moms are still getting paid less.
- ▶ And yet, society still expects us to "do it all."

Cool, cool, cool.

Many moms feel like they have to juggle multiple jobs just to keep their families afloat, all while being expected to manage the home, handle childcare (which costs more than a mortgage in some places), and still somehow prioritize their health and well-being.

This financial strain is brutally *crushing*. It forces moms into an impossible situation where self-care, personal growth, and even rest become luxuries they can't afford.

And let's not forget the invisible costs of motherhood, the unpaid labor that never gets factored into salaries or financial statements. The emotional load of keeping track of doctor's appointments, meal planning, birthday celebrations, managing tantrums, cleaning, scheduling playdates, and the *thousand* other mental tabs open at all times. Moms are basically running multi-million dollar operations without so much as a paycheck.

The solution? We need to stop accepting financial inequality as "just the way it is." We need *real* support. Paid leave, affordable childcare, fair wages, and an economy that recognizes the *actual* cost of raising the next generation.

Until then? Moms are out here performing economic miracles every single day, and *that* deserves some serious respect.

Burnout: The Unspoken Epidemic

Let's get one thing straight: motherhood should not feel like an unpaid, overworked CEO position. But that's exactly what it has become.

Between the financial stress, mental load, and relentless expectations, moms are carrying more weight than ever before. And what happens when you're constantly overworked, undervalued, and running on stress? Burnout.

Burnout isn't just "being tired." It's chronic, soul-sucking exhaustion that seeps into every aspect of life:

▶ Your body starts to breaking down—constant colds, headaches, digestive issues, random body aches.

▶ Your brain turns to mush—brain fog, forgetfulness, zero motivation.

▶ Your emotions are fried—irritability, depression, anxiety, no patience left for even the smallest inconveniences.

▶ Your relationships suffer—your partner, your kids, your friendships all feel like too much.

And it's not just emotional. Burnout wreaks havoc physically, too:

▶ **Cortisol levels skyrocket** – Your body is stuck in survival mode, which can lead to weight gain, blood sugar imbalances, and a sluggish metabolism.

▶ **The immune system tanks** – Burnout depletes your body's ability to fight off illness, leaving you constantly sick and run down.

▶ **Increased risk of serious health conditions** – Chronic stress is directly linked to heart disease, high blood pressure, and autoimmune disorders.

And yet, **moms are still expected to keep going**. There's no real safety net, no built-in recovery period. The world doesn't stop when we burn out. It just *expects us to keep functioning anyway.*

Personal Time? Hahaha

Because, apparently, self-care is for people who don't have kids.

Motherhood is the art of putting everyone else first while our own needs get kicked to the curb. This self-sacrificial approach, while rooted in love and dedication, is a surefire way to burn out and lose our sanity. The more we prioritize everything and everyone else, the further we slip into exhaustion, loneliness, and self-neglect. We end up too tired to keep up with friendships, have zero interest in sex, eat like we're on a junk food rollercoaster, and start believing we're failing at everything.

Finding time for anything that resembles leisure, hobbies, or even simple relaxation is a Herculean task for moms. And ironically, the mere idea of planning "me time" can give us anxiety. Balancing work, household duties, and childcare leaves us with about as much personal time as a snowball in hell. The result? Stress levels spike, and we feel like isolated hermits, disconnected from the world beyond our endless to-do lists.

On top of all the visible tasks we perform, we also carry the mental load of the family. We're the ones planning, organizing, and remembering all the little things that keep the household from falling apart. This invisible labor is mentally and emotionally draining. And guess what? It often goes unrecognized and unappreciated. Just think about what happens when mom goes out of town for the weekend—chaos erupts, and everyone is desperate for her to come back. Yet, when she's around, a simple "thank you" is as rare as a mermaid sighting.

Dr. Sheryl Ziegler, a Denver-based psychologist, has spent years observing moms suffering from the strains of parenthood. She consistently finds that burnout is reinforced by feelings of guilt, shame, and loneliness. "Mothers who over-involve themselves gradually become overwhelmed by perceived pressures and end up blaming themselves instead of their situations. So, we become both the victims and the perpetrators." Seriously, that totally sucks!

Ziegler notes that today's families lack the freedoms we, and our parents, once had. In my childhood, kids were told to go outside and not come back until it was dark. Now, we're all about flashcards and structured playdates. We've taken on the roles of playmates, coaches, and entertainment directors—along with the mile long list of every other role. These are WAY too many responsibilities for any one person to carry.

And let's not forget the shift in expectations around household chores. Many moms take on the overwhelming majority of household labor and don't even expect their kids to pick up after themselves. This further fuels our feelings of overwhelm and burnout. So, here we are, juggling all these responsibilities with no end in sight and very little impactful help.

The **stress moms carry daily** is basically the parenting equivalent of scaling Mt. Everest (except no one hands you oxygen, there's no base camp to rest, and your sherpa–aka coffee–is barely keeping you alive). 25% of women under the age of 24 report anxiety and depression, in comparison to their mothers in the 1990s who only reported 17%. The longer we push through without support, the more exhausting and suffocating the climb feels. Honestly, where's the damn rescue helicopter when we need it?!

CHAPTER 03

After All That Chaos: Let's Redeem Your Peace of Mind

If you made it through Chapter 2 without throwing your phone across the room or scream-laughing into a laundry pile, congrats—you're already stronger than you think. We unpacked the emotional circus that is the modern mom's brain: the mental load, the invisible labor, the constant juggling act that leaves us wondering when exactly we became the unpaid CEO of a 24/7 household startup. And if it felt like a lot, that's because it is. Being a mom in today's world isn't just a job—it's an Olympic-level sport with no coach, no halftime, and definitely no trophies.

So now that we've aired out the chaos, let's talk about something else: **hope**. Yes, it still exists. And no, it doesn't require a 3-week spa retreat or a trust fund. It starts with something simpler. Smaller. Something you can do in your kitchen, your

23

car, even while hiding in the bathroom for a five-minute breather.

One of the easiest and most effective ways I've found to start rebuilding peace in the middle of the madness? **Somatic healing.**

Wait—before your brain jumps to a dramatic mental image of incense, gongs, or interpretive dance (though hey, no judgment if that's your thing), hear me out. Somatic healing isn't some far-off concept for people with too much free time. It's a grounded, practical, body-based approach to resetting your nervous system—one you can work into even the most chaotic of mom schedules.

So... What Is Somatic Healing?

Somatic healing is a form of mind-body therapy rooted in the idea that trauma, stress, and emotion don't just live in our heads—they live in our bodies, too. Think of it like emotional housekeeping. Instead of letting all that stress collect like dust in your muscles and nerves, somatic healing helps you clean it out through movement, breath, body awareness, and mindfulness. You don't have to "fix" everything. You just have to start *feeling* again.

Sound intimidating? It's not. This isn't about adding another thing to your to-do list. This is about subtracting what no longer serves you—especially the pressure to carry the mental load of the whole damn family without breaking a sweat.

Why Moms Need Somatic Healing Now More Than Ever

Let's connect the dots: the mental load we talked about in Chapter 2? That sh*t is heavy. All those invisible tasks, emotional check-ins, meal plans, diaper bags, drop-offs, work emails, playdates, and permission slips… they don't just disappear. They live in your body. In your tight shoulders. In your clenched jaw. In that racing heart and that gnawing pit in your stomach.

Your body is keeping score. And it's asking for a timeout.

Somatic healing is how you *take back the remote* from the chaos and hit "pause." It's not about running away from your life, it's about running toward yourself again.

SOMATIC HEALING CAN

Reduces stress and anxiety

Simple practices like progressive muscle relaxation and deep breathing release tension and lower stress levels.

Enhances emotional regulation

Helps you process emotions in real-time before they become overwhelming.

Improves cognitive function

Movement-based therapies like yoga or tai chi strengthen neural pathways, boosting memory and mental clarity.

Promotes better sleep

Relaxation techniques help regulate sleep cycles, making it easier to rest deeply.

Boosts overall well-being

Strengthens the mind-body connection, leaving you feeling more grounded and in control of your health.

How You Can Actually Do This (Without Losing Your Mind)

You don't need a yoga studio or a silent mountain retreat. You just need a few simple tools to get back into your body—because peace doesn't come from doing more. It comes from doing less, more intentionally.

Here are just a few ways you can start:

► **Body Scans** while lying next to your kid at bedtime. Check in with yourself by mentally scanning your body for areas of tension or discomfort.

► **Deep belly breathing** in the school pickup line. Deep belly breathing or alternate nostril breathing can instantly calm your nervous system.

► **Stretching or light movement** during nap time. Gentle movement paired with focused breathing helps reset your stress response.

► **Shaking it out** (yes, literally shaking your arms, legs, hips) when your energy feels stuck.

► **Placing a hand on your heart** when your brain starts spiraling. This helps you focus on a specific area, to take a "pause", and get back to a calmer rhythm.

It's all about micro-moments. You don't have to wait until you have time—you just need to take a moment, as you are, where you are.

CHAPTER 04

How the Mental Health System Has Failed Women

Let's talk about mental health for moms. Or rather, let's talk about how, for decades, no one really gave a crap about it. In the '80s, if you were a woman struggling mentally, you had two choices: suffer in silence, or get slapped with a prescription-that may or may not work, but would absolutely screw with your body even more.

Postpartum depression? No such thing in the 80's. Not officially, anyway. If you admitted to feeling exhausted, overwhelmed, or (God forbid) like you weren't the glowing, joyful mother you were supposed to be, you were labeled "hormonal", "weak", or "hysterical". The go-to solution? Medicate her. Sedate her. Numb her. But never, ever listen to her.

And that's exactly what happened to my mom.

HOW MY MOM BECAME AN EXPERIMENT OF THE 1980S MENTAL HEALTH SYSTEM

My mom was diagnosed with severe depression in her 30s, shortly after having her sixth child. Now, knowing what I know today, I'd bet good money that she was experiencing postpartum depression. Something that wasn't even on the medical community's radar back then. The idea that a mother could love her child but still struggle mentally? Unheard of. Instead of recognizing the very real hormonal, emotional, and societal pressures weighing on new moms, the mental health industry did what it always did: diagnose first, ask questions never.

She was given a bipolar, manic depressive disorder diagnosis. Not because it was necessarily correct, but because doctors didn't have the research, training, or frankly, the interest in studying women's mental health enough to make an informed decision. And what do you do with a fresh diagnosis in the '80s? You get loaded up on psychiatric meds that make you feel like a walking ghost. And then you become part of the grand experiment.

The mental health industry was understaffed, underfunded, and completely clueless about how to handle women's mental health struggles. My mom's case? A textbook example of how women became lab rats. What followed was years of heavy medication, weight gain, and worsening mental fog. Every time she felt awful from the side effects, the answer was always the same:

"Here's another prescription."

At one point, things got so bad that she underwent electric shock therapy for a year and a half.

Electric. Shock. Therapy.

In an era when they barely understood mental health to begin with, let alone women's mental health.

Did it help? Not really.

What it did do was leave her with long-term memory issues that still affect her today. And as if that wasn't enough, she was also left with long-term physical damage from these medications.

Because here's the thing Big Pharma won't tell you: long-term use of psychiatric medications can have devastating effects on your body. And my mom is living proof. She was on decades' worth of medications. Ones that have been found to be linked to cognitive decline, neurological issues, and even bone density loss. So when she was diagnosed with osteopenia, was it just bad luck? Hell no. I'd bet everything that the same medications prescribed to "help" her mental health also contributed to breaking down her physical health. (Not that we can prove that , because like I stated before, there are basically zero studies on the health of mothers in the realm of psychiatric drugs.)

And guess what? This isn't rare.

Many of these psychiatric drugs—especially antidepressants, antipsychotics, and mood stabilizers—have been proven to have a negative impact on women's health. They interfere with calcium absorption, disrupt hormonal balance, and can even accelerate osteoporosis.

So while my mom was just trying to survive, the very drugs that were meant to "help" her were silently setting her up for a future of physical pain and fragility.

And yet, no one warned her. No one questioned it. No one cared.

Fast forward to today, and women's mental health is still an afterthought. Sure, the diagnoses have gotten stronger, and there's at least an acknowledgment that postpartum depression exists, but has treatment actually improved?

Not really.

Instead of getting to the root of mental health struggles, we're still being handed a one-size-fits-all pharmaceutical answer. More prescriptions have been developed, but minimal research has been done in holistic or alternative treatments.

- ► Where are the studies on how food affects neurotransmitters?
- ► Where is the investment in therapy accessibility over medication dependency?
- ► Why is it that the moment a woman struggles, the automatic response is a script instead of a support system?

This isn't to say medication doesn't have its place. It absolutely does. But it shouldn't be the only tool in the toolbox.

And yet, here we are.

How My Mom Took Her Health Back

After decades of being told to just "trust the process" while still feeling like crap, my mom finally had enough. She started questioning everything. What was actually helping? What was just masking symptoms? What was actively making her feel worse?

With my guidance and help of her psychiatrist (one of the rare ones who actually listened), she made the terrifying decision to start tapering off some of the medications that were clouding her mind.

She began exploring alternative healing.

- ▶ She changed her diet to support her brain health.
- ▶ She prioritized exercise to help regulate her mood.
- ▶ She used acupuncture to relieve stress and pain.
- ▶ She focused on supplements that supported her nervous system.
- ▶ She practiced stress management techniques that helped her heal from years of emotional and physical strain.

And for the first time in years, she felt like herself again. She was clear-headed, empowered, and in control. She put in the hard work, with some guidance and help from me, and changed the outcome of her story.

My mom's journey isn't unique. It's the story of so many women who have been misdiagnosed, overmedicated, and left feeling like they were broken. When, in reality, the system was broken, not them.

It's a story about how women's mental health has been ignored for far too long and how, even today, the system still fails to offer real solutions beyond pills.

It's a story about resilience, self-advocacy, and the power of taking control of your own well-being.

And it's a reminder that while we can't change the past, we sure as hell can change how we approach mental health moving forward.

Because women deserve better. And it starts with demanding better.

CHAPTER 05

Moms Are Powerful, Don't Mess With Them

A mom's love is like the ultimate superpower, quietly shaping our kids in ways we can't even fully grasp. We're the emotional glue that keeps them stable, the cheerleaders boosting their self-esteem, and the launchpad for their curiosity.

We're also the ones teaching them to manage those inevitable meltdowns and navigate life's roller coasters. We're instilling values such as empathy, compassion, and the difference between right and wrong–basically fine-tuning their moral compass.

And let's not forget, our love turns them into leaders. We're showing our kids how to demand their rightful seat at life's table, helping them build the emotional muscle they need to be happy, satisfied, and well-adjusted adults.

MOMS LEAD BY EXAMPLE

We lead by example in every part of our kids' lives, whether it's fighting for their health, teaching them resilience, or showing them how to trust themselves. That's why **research** shows that kids raised by strong, determined mothers grow up to be confident leaders. Moms don't just shape their children, we shape the future. If there is anything we can learn from our own personal experiences as moms, it's that our instincts are often more powerful than any degree, diagnosis, or dismissal.

Interpersonal Effectiveness

Moms are pros at listening and sharing, translating into boss-level communication skills for happy, healthy members of society. We're all about those heart-to-heart talks that build trust and understanding in the family — skills every child needs in their toolkit.

Emotional Intelligence And Compassion

Moms teach their children to express their feelings and show empathy for others. When kids incorporate these qualities into their lives, they can foster a more positive and productive environment that extends into adulthood.

Patience

Moms pretty much invented patience. Whether we're helping spell "cat" for the umpteenth time or teaching our kids to drive as soon as they get that learning permit, we've got the patience of saints. Children and adults who can stay calm under pressure and keep their eyes on the prize are set up for success.

Time Management

Juggling multiple tasks effectively is something mothers do instinctively. We're masters of the calendar when balancing work deadlines with carpooling and after school activities— and all the pep talks along the way. As our kids get older, the ability to prioritize tasks and manage time efficiently is critical.

Adaptability

Moms are constantly rolling with the punches, whether it's a last-minute change of plans or a surprise visit from a long-lost relative. We stay ready to pivot immediately—an essential trait in today's fast-paced world that our kids can take with them when they leave the nest.

Resilience

Moms are superheroes when it comes to bouncing back from setbacks. We handle challenges like champs, powering through tough times and keeping the family morale high. We are also graceful in admitting mistakes and learning from failures. Our kids will need this same resilience to navigate the ups and downs of life, from squabbles on the playground to conflict with partners and colleagues.

Crisis Management

We are masters of keeping our cool when chaos strikes. Whether it's a scraped knee or de-escalating our kids' full-blown meltdowns in public, we stealthily navigate these emotionally charged situations. As moms, we have to be able to make quick, intelligent decisions when the pressure is on and our kids benefit from watching us do just that.

> **Negotiation Skills**
> Whether brokering peace between screeching siblings or haggling over curfew times, mothers are negotiating wizards. These skills are invaluable in almost all of life's situations.

But, being Mom isn't just about teaching lessons and setting rules. It's about trusting ourselves. Because if there's one thing I've learned, it's this: *Moms always know best.*

When a Mother's Instinct Becomes the Lifeline

It was a Thursday morning in January 2017, my daughter Izzie got sick. It seemed like a simple case of strep throat—fever, a lump on her throat, and discomfort while swallowing. Her pediatrician diagnosed her with strep, even though the office test came back negative. But, hey, doctors know best, right? He started her on antibiotics "just in case."

Within 24 hours, Izzie's fever roared back. This time, she had a rash on her arms, chest, and upper thighs. Her eyes turned an alarming shade of red, and the lump on her throat swelled dramatically.

This was not strep. Something was clearly wrong. And when something is wrong, you don't wait for permission to act. With my husband out running errands, I made the call: we're going to Urgent Care.

By some divine intervention, the doctor we saw happened to be a pediatric cardiologist. Within two minutes, she looked at Izzie and said a word I had never heard before:

"This is Kawasaki Disease."

Kawasaki? The only association I had with that word was motorcycles. This was something entirely different. The doctor handed me an information sheet and said:

"You need to take her to the ER immediately."

Cue full-on mom panic. But, as any mom will tell you, panic is a luxury we don't have when our kids need us.

Despite the pediatric cardiologist's note, the ER staff acted like Izzie had nothing more than a stubborn fever. They gave her Motrin, watched her fever drop, and sent us home with more antibiotics.

I wanted to scream. I knew this was not just a fever. I told them about the diagnosis, the symptoms, the fact that something was seriously wrong. But they dismissed it. Because that's what happens to moms all the time. Even when we bring them evidence, even when we lay out the facts, we are ignored, told we are crazy, and that we don't know what we are talking about– just "trust the experts!"

A Mother's Instinct is the Best Medical Degree in the World

By Saturday morning, Izzie was worse. Her fever hit 104, her rash spread, her tongue swelled to the size of a strawberry, and her eyes burned bright red.

Enough.

I took her back to her pediatrician, who immediately confirmed the Kawasaki Disease diagnosis. He wrote a detailed note for the ER and handed me his personal cell number. "If they push back again, call me," he said.

This time, armed with a doctor's orders and a mama bear's rage, we went back to the ER and demanded action. Finally, they admitted her. She started IVIG treatments that night. But the road to recovery was anything but smooth.

By Wednesday, her condition barely improved. A specialist suggested she had something even rarer than KD, and suddenly, Izzie was placed in quarantine. And yet, I knew. I knew the original doctor was right. I knew we were dealing with Kawasaki.

That night, the on-call doctor strode in, locked eyes with me, and (with the unwavering confidence of someone who had been through the trenches of motherhood herself) declared without hesitation, "We'll take his advice cautiously, but I'm starting the second round of IVIG tonight. Is that okay, Mrs. Steele?" It was like the mama bear in her wanted to rage as much as I did against the disease specialist.

Damn right, it was okay.

I nodded. We went into full battle mode. And by Thursday afternoon, Izzie's fever broke. Her rash disappeared. And for the first time in days, she had enough energy to eat. She was on the mend. Days later, the disease specialist's tests came back negative. The original diagnosis was correct all along. (Insert massive eye roll here.)

Why Moms Never Retreat

Looking back, I'm grateful. Grateful for the doctor who caught it early. Grateful that I trusted my gut. Grateful that I never backed down. Because if I had listened to the ER the first time and "waited it out"? I don't even want to think about what could have happened.

Today, Izzie is thriving. She's the most chill, kindhearted kid you'll ever meet. I like to think that her journey taught her something about resilience and the power of listening to your gut. If nothing else, it reinforced one unshakable truth: Moms just know. And we will never stop fighting for our kids.

When a mom says something is wrong, listen.

When a mom pushes for an answer, take her seriously

When a mom demands better, don't stand in her way.

Because we always, always know best.

Izzie's story isn't one of a kind. Moms everywhere are fighting to be heard in the medical system, in their own homes, and even in their own minds. We've been taught to doubt ourselves, to accept dismissive doctors, and to put everyone else's needs before our own. But no more.

The healthcare system wasn't built to prioritize moms, it was built to keep us running just well enough to keep doing everything for everyone else. But if we're going to change the game, we need to stop playing by their rules.

What you will learn throughout this book is how to take back your power, advocate for better healthcare, and ensure you never, ever get ignored again. Motherhood doesn't have to mean sacrificing your well-being. Taking small steps to prioritize yourself isn't selfish, it's survival. And when moms are thriving, the whole family benefits. It's time to take our health back, one simple step at a time.

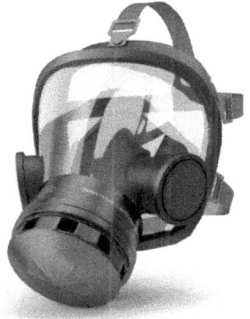

CHAPTER 06

F*ck Pharma

D id you know that marketing pharmaceuticals directly to consumers is only legal in the United States and New Zealand? Yep, everywhere else, it's banned. This loophole lets Big Pharma tug at our deepest fears (of suffering, of death) just to stuff their pockets, and they're doing it all with the blessing of the United States government.

Dr. Dee Mangin, associate professor at the Christchurch School of Medicine and Health Sciences in New Zealand, nailed it in an interview with the World Health Organization:

> "The truth is direct-to-consumer advertising is used to drive choice rather than inform it... the 'driving' is typically in the direction of expensive brand-name drugs. Consumers then go to their doctors, and the pressure to prescribe begins."

Pharmaceutical companies are on a never-ending profit hunt, and their golden goose? Pills. If there's no consumer demand, there's no business. Simple as that.

That's why **over 20% of U.S. adults aged 40 and older are on five or more prescription drugs.** (Stop, and read that again!) Big Pharma has turned this into a gold mine, preying on fear, chronic illness, and utilizing a medical system designed to manage disease rather than prevent or cure it.

How Pharma Keeps You Hooked

Meet the "disease mongers". A term science writer Lynne Payer coined to describe Big Pharma and its unofficial hype squad, including doctors and insurers. These folks have mastered the art of convincing perfectly healthy people that they're sick, or that mildly sick people are on death's doorstep. And it works. Just take a look at how diagnostic benchmarks keep getting lowered to make more people eligible for medication (hello, "prehypertension" and "pre-diabetes").

Pharma's biggest flex isn't just convincing you that you're sick. It's keeping you hooked once they do.

Take Eli Lilly, for example. When Prozac's patent was about to expire, they played a dirty trick. They rebranded it as Sarafem, convinced the FDA that PMDD (Pre-Menstrual Dysphoric Disorder) was a catastrophic disease. Big Pharma didn't just invent a disease to keep profits rolling in, they rebranded an old drug and charged people more for it in the process.

This is what we're up against.

Feeling a bit angry yet? **You should be**.

Cancer is a huge one for women. What Pharma doesn't want you to know, is many cancers are preventable (and many times reversible) through lifestyle choices, and holistic or alternative practices. For many women, those options are never even discussed, or presented as options. Take my cousin, for example.

She was the embodiment of energy and ambition. A new mom, thriving in Nashville's food and beverage industry, juggling the chaos of motherhood while running two new bars—one of which earned her and her husband a feature in a well-known Food & Wine magazine. Life was on fire.

And then cancer happened.

Stage 4 breast cancer. In her 30s. With a baby boy at home.

She did what any mother would do: she fought like hell. She put nursing on pause, dove into chemo, and leaned on her Nashville community—a city known for its big hearts and even bigger support networks. But my cousin wasn't just fighting—she was documenting the battle with her trademark sarcastic humor (must run in the family).

She launched a Facebook blog called "Positively Cancer," where she shared the ugly, the funny, and the brutally honest truth about what cancer does to you. She made people laugh, cry, and—most importantly…think. She showed thousands of people that you may lose your hair, but you don't have to lose your resiliency or sense of humor.

But here's the thing: Cancer didn't kill her. The complications from chemo did.

My cousin did everything she was "supposed" to do. She followed the protocol. She fought with everything she had. She endured a double mastectomy. Then, chemo-induced cysts in her uterus meant she had to have a hysterectomy–a crushing blow for her and her husband, who had dreamed of more kids.

And in the end? A virus entered her spinal fluid during a procedure and traveled to her brain. Her immune system, obliterated by treatment, couldn't fight it off.

This is the part that haunts me.

This isn't an anti-chemo manifesto. This is a wake-up call. A reminder that medicine should be a strategy, not a blindfolded game of Russian Roulette.

My cousin didn't have a choice. When you're in Stage 4, you don't get to "explore your options." But if I could turn back time, I'd wonder: could holistic approaches have improved her odds? Could integrative medicine have mitigated some of the collateral damage? Could supporting her immune system alongside the treatment have given her more time?

Here's what I do know: Mindset matters. Immensely. My cousin proved that every single day.

Despite the hell she was going through, she chose positivity, humor, and strength. She faced death with the kind of grace and grit that most people don't have on their best days. And that's what I want people to take from her story. Not just the heartbreak, but the reminder that how you fight matters.

This isn't just about cancer. This is about demanding better. Better research, better options, better care. Because right now?

The system isn't built to save you. It's built to profit off you, and if you die in the process, oh well.

The Business of Keeping You Sick

Another classic Pharma move? Tweaking the rules for diagnosing diseases.

Dr. Adriane Fugh-Berman, head of the industry watchdog group PharmedOut.org at Georgetown, pointed out how the benchmarks for diagnosing conditions like diabetes and high cholesterol have conveniently been lowered over time.

> "The very numbers we use have been reduced to the point of absurdity," she said. "120/80 used to be normal blood pressure; now it's 'prehypertension.'" And no, it's not because science has advanced.

Ray Moynihan, an Australia-based journalist and disease-mongering researcher, presents it this way in his book *Selling Sickness*:

> "We're in this crazy paradox where we're technically healthier than ever, but somehow we think we're sicker and sicker. Minor symptoms, everyday annoyances, aging, and just being human are all getting labeled as medical conditions."

It's like we're living in a medical drama where every little inconvenience is a full-blown crisis.

On a side note, no other medical specialty has turned more of life's everyday quirks into full-blown diagnoses than psychiatry. And guess what? No other specialty is quite as snug with Big Pharma. They've got a well-oiled machine of conference sponsorships, CME funding, research grants, and donations to patient advocacy groups. Those groups, ever so grateful for the cash, are all too happy to endorse the latest drug if it promises to "help others."

How to Fight Back Against the System

Alright, now that you know how Pharma plays the game, it's time to **rewrite the rules for yourself**.

1   Question Everything – If a doctor prescribes medication, ask why. Are there **lifestyle changes** or alternative treatments that could be tried first?

2   **Find Practitioners Who Support Integrative Health** – Look for functional medicine doctors, naturopaths, and holistic nutritionists who see the whole picture.

3   **Educate Yourself on Nutrition** – Food is medicine. The right diet can reduce inflammation, balance hormones, and prevent disease. (Things drugs can only manage, and even then, usually not effectively).

4   **Build Your Own Health Team** – Seek out a mix of conventional and holistic practitioners who respect your choices.

5   **Demand Better Research and Policies** – Pharma won't change unless we demand it. Support health-focused organizations, vote for policies that promote alternative medicine, and advocate for yourself and your family.

Pharma's Business Model

In a truly healthy world, the demand for drugs would barely exist. If the system actually prioritized real health, we wouldn't need a never-ending supply of pharmaceutical interventions to keep us functioning.

And yet, here we are. One fact that's gaining quite a bit of attention is that around **80% of chronic diseases are tied to lifestyle factors**. What's on that list? Stress, diet, and exercise. Some practitioners, like those from The **Cleveland Clinic** and **Harvard**, think it's even more, upwards of 90% of chronic diseases that are linked directly to lifestyle. And no, it's not just the wellness guru who wears crystals. It's legit medical professionals.

Instead of tackling the root causes of health problems, doctors are practically handing out prescriptions as if it's halloween, and patients are happily munching them down, not knowing the consequences. The top pills in America? They're all about managing cholesterol, blood pressure, and endocrine disorders. (Surprise, surprise!) And, Pharma's self-regulation? Let's just say it's about as reliable as a screen door on a submarine. Seriously, we're supposed to trust these guys with our health and well-being? You've probably heard about the opioid crisis, but that's just the tip of the iceberg. Think about all the recalls, financial settlements, and questionable products they've shoved down our throats. These pharmaceutical giants seem to have a knack for selling first and asking questions later. Just look at Johnson & Johnson, GlaxoSmithKline, and Pfizer—**they've all shelled out billions** for "off-label promotion," which basically means they've been caught prescribing drugs for uses they weren't approved for.

And then **there are the recalls**. Remember Merck's Vioxx or Pfizer's Bextra? These were supposed to be top-tier treatments, but they turned out to be minorly better than your average over-the-counter meds. And just for good measure, **about 1,279 drugs get recalled every year**. Clearly, the industry hasn't exactly been taking its punches to heart. With pharma companies, there's no incentive to actually keep you healthy. Once a disease is "cured," the cash flow dries up. *They're not in the health business; they're in the disease management business, plain and simple.*

Here's some numbers that will make you nauseated:

In 2023, opioids were involved in **81,083 overdose deaths,** according to the CDC—a ten-fold increase from 1999.

222 people in the U.S. die daily from opioid overdoses. Yet, private insurers happily cover addictive drugs over natural, effective alternatives for pain management.

1 in 10 women between **18 and 39 are on antidepressants**. That number jumps to 1 in 5 for women aged 40 to 59, and 1 in 4 for women over 60. Women are prescribed these drugs at a much higher rate than men.

And the kicker? Many of these prescriptions women are taking have never been tested on women. Women account for only 30% of participants in cardiovascular research, despite heart disease being a leading cause of death for women. So, here we are, buried under a mountain of medication, still feeling miserable. Maybe it's time to push back and demand something better than just more pills.

CHAPTER 07

Integrative Medicine vs. Big Pharma

This is where I introduce you to Integrative Medicine as it is becoming quite the hot topic in the health field lately. Think of integrative medicine as the friend who's brutally honest with you. No sugarcoating, just the truth. She tells you what you don't want to hear. This modality is all about getting to the root cause of your issues and treating symptoms, like pain or high blood pressure, only when absolutely necessary. First, it explores safer, natural therapies because who needs those nasty side effects if they can be avoided? While synthetic drugs just slap a Band-Aid on the problem, integrative medicine is all about supporting your body to stay in tip-top shape using natural therapies and supplements. It's like the anti-Big Pharma. Or the oddball cousin of conventional medicine.

For starters, the initial consultation with a naturopath or functional medicine doctor will run you between an hour to an hour and a half. In a conventional doctor's office? You're lucky if you lay eyes on your doctor for more than 10 minutes. But, apparently that's long enough to be diagnosed and sent off with a hastily written prescription .

But picture this: What if doctors actually took a moment to help patients change their lifestyles, and provided some genuine support before handing out those meds? This is where Integrative healthcare enters the chat.

If enough of us decided to tackle lifestyle changes, we could see diseases start to vanish instead of just getting managed with a med menu. That's why I'm so fired up about health and wellness for moms. We're on the front lines of healthcare for ourselves and our families, which puts us in a prime position to demand some changes, and refuse to settle for pills as the only answer.

Just like my cousin and my mom so deserved. And so do you.

What is Integrative Health and Functional Medicine?

Integrative and functional medicine are the rockstars of healthcare. They take a whole-person approach, looking at all aspects of a mom's life and combining conventional, traditional, and evidence-based therapies. (Hence the hour-plus initial visit.)

This approach is especially useful for preventing disease, and treating chronic conditions like depression, diabetes, and autoimmune disorders, which are heavily influenced by diet and lifestyle.

INTEGRATIVE MEDICINE FOCUSES ON:

Nutrition (because food is medicine)

Exercise (movement is essential for health)

Stress management (less stress, fewer symptoms)

Sleep (better sleep = better health)

Holistic treatments like acupuncture, massage, and herbal therapy.

Can you imagine hearing a doctor prescribe you a massage?! Sign me up!

Natural, Less Invasive Treatments? Yes, Please!

Sure, prescription medications are sometimes necessary, but they're not always the perfect solution.

For quite a few years, I was on hormone replacement therapies (HRTs) through my naturopath, until my levels balanced out with the help of structural lifestyle changes. But we need to understand that prescriptions can be ineffective, or come with serious side effects—which in most cases leads to more prescriptions. It's like a domino effect.

Integrative medicine offers natural approaches for tackling health concerns, emphasizing minimally invasive treatments whenever possible. Think of it as the love child of conventional and complementary medicine. (And no, I am NOT saying a diet of oranges cures cancer.) What I *am* saying is it combines traditional methods with safe, evidence-based alternatives, while boosting your body's innate ability to heal. As you optimize your diet and lifestyle, you often end up needing fewer meds. Imagine that!

In her New York Times Best Selling book, *Good Energy*, Dr. Casey Means discusses how many chronic illnesses share a common origin: metabolic dysfunction. She uses the metaphor of a tree: The trunk represents metabolic dysfunction. The branches are chronic diseases like Type 2 diabetes, obesity, and cancer.

Much like a tree that becomes diseased through lack of water, sunlight, or healthy soil, humans develop disease when their environment and lifestyle are out of balance—poor diet, sleep deprivation, chronic stress, and sedentary habits accelerate metabolic dysfunction. We have to nurture our bodies with good energy to maintain our health just like a tree needs optimal soil, sunlight, and water.

How Integrative Medicine Works

- ▶ **Health and Well-being, Not Just Sicknes**s – Focuses on prevention and longevity vs managing symptoms.

- ▶ **Treating the Whole You, Not Just a Symptom** – Assesses the full picture: biological, behavioral, psychosocial, and environmental factors.

- ▶ **Root Causes, Not Just Band-Aids** – Seeks to identify and address the actual cause of disease.

- ▶ **Personalized Just for You** – No one-size-fits-all approach. Treatments are customized to each patient.

- ▶ **Incorporating Eastern Wisdom** – Uses herbs, botanicals, acupuncture, and ancient healing methods in conjunction with modern science.

Functional Medicine:
Actually Finding the Root Cause

This is why **functional medicine** is on the rise. People (especially moms) are **done with** the one-size-fits-all, take-this-pill-and-go-away- approach to health.

Take my friend, for example. For years, she struggled with bloating, gas, diarrhea, and gut issues that no doctor could explain. It started in childhood. Random stomach pains that were brushed off as stress or bad food choices. The solution? A bottle of Pepto, a pat on the back, and a "you'll be fine."

Fast-forward to adulthood, and the symptoms didn't magically disappear. By the time she hit her early 30s, she knew something was off, because at a certain point, living in constant discomfort and praying you won't have to run to the nearest bathroom isn't normal.

She did exactly what most of us would do: went to a general practitioner.

Tests were run. A food sensitivity test came back with vague answers. She was referred to a GI specialist. Got handed a prescription to take "when her stomach hurt" (oh, how thoughtful). Got told to follow a Low FODMAP diet (which, as a vegetarian, was nearly impossible). And when none of that worked? The doctor suggested a colonoscopy. At this point, she had enough.

Why was she being shuffled between specialists without anyone actually trying to figure out what was going on? Why was she being given pills to "manage" symptoms instead of being told how to heal?

So she did something most people don't think to do: she stopped playing along with the conventional healthcare game. We had some in depth conversations, and she approached her health from a new perspective. She ditched the traditional doctors and started exploring functional medicine. She met with naturopaths who actually listened to her. She discovered that her gut issues weren't random, they were connected to stress, diet, gut bacteria imbalances, and inflammation. She found out that her SIBO (Small Intestinal Bacterial Overgrowth), candida overgrowth, and leaky gut weren't just things she had to live with. For the first time, she wasn't being told to "just take something when it flares up"–she was being given real strategies to heal. Through a nutritional plan structured for her, supplements that targeted specific deficiencies into balance, as well as a couple of procedures that would impact her health in the long run, she was on her way to feeling "herself" again.

Functional medicine asks the real questions:

WHY are you inflamed?

WHAT is triggering your symptoms?

HOW can you actually heal?

Instead of masking symptoms, **functional medicine practitioners** focus on diet, stress, gut health, sleep, and overall lifestyle changes. It's not about replacing prescriptions with supplements, it's about fixing what's broken.

And shocker? It works.

I've seen it work not just for my friend, but for myself, and many others I have assisted. Because the truth is, so many of us are walking around in survival mode. We're exhausted, emotionally drained, and stuck in a cycle of burnout, but we just assume this is how it's supposed to be.

Let's check in for a second:

Do any of these sound familiar?

Extreme fatigue? Does your burnout leave you beyond exhausted?

Feel like a bad mom? Guilt and inadequacy? Check.

Mom rage? Wild mood swings and irritability? Yep.

Feeling emotionally depleted? Numbness, disconnection, or struggling to find joy?

Limited patience? Snapping at everything and everyone?

The thing is, you don't have to feel like this.

And if you're nodding along to most of these questions, conventional medicine will probably tell you it's just "normal." They'll say it's stress. They'll offer you an antidepressant. They'll tell you to "get more sleep."

But I know firsthand it doesn't have to be this way.

Walking away from the prescription-first mentality and working with professionals who saw me as a whole person (not just a walking co-pay) was the best decision ever.

Functional medicine gave me my life back.

It did the same for my friend. And it can do the same for you.

Functional medicine physician, **Dr. Will Cole,** shares this comparison.

FUNCTIONAL MEDICINE VS. CONVENTIONAL MEDICINE	
Functional Medicine	**Conventional Medicine**
Investigate It treats symptoms by addressing the underlying cause of the problem, which leads to more profound and longer lasting results.	**Superficial** Masks or suppresses symptoms, but does not address underlying cause, which creates "patients for life".
Holistic Treats the body as an interconnected whole, and recognizes the importance of these connections in health and disease.	**Dualistic** Views the body as a collection of separate parts, each of which has its own doctor (i.e. cardiologist, podiatrist, etc.)
Safe Treatments have mild or no side effects, and other unrelated complaints often improve spontaneously.	**Side Effects** Treatments can have side effects and complications.
Patient-centered Treats the patient, not the disease. Treatments are highly individualized based on patient needs.	**Disease-centered** Treats the disease, not the patient. Patients with the same disease get the same treatment, regardless of their differences.
Participatory Patient is respected, empowered, educated and encouraged to play an active role in the healing process.	**Autocratic** Patient's opinion is often discounted or ignored, little time is spent on education, and patient may be discouraged from playing active role.
Interrogative Combines the best of both modern and traditional medicines and emphasizes importance of diet and lifestyle.	**Limited** Relies almost exclusively on drugs and surgery, in spite of their risks and complications.

FUNCTIONAL MEDICINE VS. CONVENTIONAL MEDICINE

Restorative
Tests and treatments designed to promote optimal function, prevent and reverse disease, and improve quality of life.

Palliative
Tests and treatments designed to prevent death and manage serious disease, without dealing with the underlying cause.

Preventative
Guided by the Hippocrates, the father of medicine's, saying to "let food be thy medicine, and medicine thy food".

Reactive
Focused on managing disease after it has already reached an irreversible state.

Evidence-based
Based on the latest research from peer-reviewed medical journals, and uncorrupted by corporate and political interests.

Profit-driven
Heavily influenced by profit-driven pharmaceutical and insurance companies.

Why Should You Care About Any of This?

Chronic diseases are the leading contributors to the nation's $4.1 trillion annual healthcare costs.

Most people suffering from these conditions turn to conventional medicine, which focuses on treating symptoms with pharmaceuticals or surgery. This symptom-based approach leads to dependency on drugs, because when the medication is stopped, the symptoms return. Which works well in favor of Pharma companies—but not for your health, sanity, or bank account.

We've been taught to trust a system that profits off our sickness. That doesn't mean we have to keep playing along.

CHAPTER 08

Nutrition, Movement, and Sleep

When it comes to feeling good, what you eat, how you move, and how well you sleep determine everything. I consider these the Holy Trinity of health. Nutrition fuels your energy, movement keeps your body functioning optimally, and sleep repairs and restores it all. These three pillars are inseparably linked. Mess with one, and the others inevitably suffer.

When your brain is fried, your body follows. The relentless stress of motherhood doesn't just deplete your mental reserves, it slowly chips away at your physical health, too. Chronic stress triggers inflammation, disrupts sleep, throws hormones into chaos, and weakens the immune system.

The demands of parenting, coupled with sleep deprivation and hormonal upheaval, can turn everyday exhaustion into full-blown burnout. And once you're running on empty, everything suffers. Your energy, your patience, your ability to function like a semi-normal human.

Motherhood, in many ways, is the ultimate physical, mental, and emotional health boot camp that never ends. Pregnancy, childbirth, and breastfeeding take a toll on the body, yet moms are spectacularly bad at prioritizing their own well-being. Lack of time and opportunity to address personal health concerns leaves many moms feeling drained, overwhelmed, and teetering on the edge of collapse.

By making small adjustments in each area, you create a positive ripple effect that transforms both mental and physical health, without adding more stress to your already maxed-out plate.

5 Small Changes That Make a Big Difference

Instead of overhauling your entire lifestyle (because who has time for that?), focus on these five simple shifts that have a major impact:

1 **Fuel Your Body with Real Food** – No, you don't need to turn into a gourmet health chef. Just focus on eating whole foods 80% of the time. Prioritize protein, healthy fats, and fiber to stabilize energy and hormones. Swap out the processed junk for real, nutrient-dense options.

2 **Prioritize Sleep (even if It feels impossible)** – Your body needs rest to function. Create a simple, realistic sleep routine: dim lights an hour before bed, limit late-night scrolling, and aim for at least one night a week of uninterrupted sleep. Even small tweaks to sleep habits can yield major benefits.

3 **Move Your Body in a Way That Feels Good** – Exercise doesn't have to be a chore. Whether it's stretching in the morning, walking with a friend, or dancing in the kitchen while making dinner, movement is medicine. Start small and build from there.

5 Small Changes That Make a Big Difference

4   **Reduce Stress with Breathwork & Mini-Resets** – You don't need an hour-long meditation to reap the benefits of stress reduction. Just a few deep belly breaths or a five-minute break from overstimulation (yes, even locking yourself in the bathroom counts!) can reset your nervous system.

5   **Hydrate Like It's Your Job** – Dehydration is your enemy - it exacerbates exhaustion, brain fog, and stress. Keep a water bottle nearby and actually drink from it throughout the day. Bonus points for adding electrolytes (without sugar!) to support energy levels.

So, let's break it down in a way that actually makes sense for moms who don't have time for BS health trends.

Nutrition: The Foundation of Health

We've all heard the saying "You are what you eat," but seriously, what does that even mean? No, it doesn't mean you'll turn into a giant carrot if you munch too many, or that eating fat will literally make you fat. What we eat is the foundation of our health–fueling our bodies, impacting our mood, and determining how well we function.

Ignoring proper nutrition is like ignoring the check engine light in your car. Keep feeding your body junk, and eventually it's going to break down. Hello, weight gain, arthritis, diabetes, and heart disease. And we all know, moms don't have time to be sick.

Here's where the fun begins: every bite you take sends a message to your body. Whole, nutrient-dense foods say, *"Hey, let's thrive!"* while ultra-processed junk says, *"Buckle up, inflammation incoming."*

As *Perspectives in Nutrition* puts it, "Nutrients are the nourishing substances in food essential for growth, development, and maintaining body functions. Essential: meaning that without them, your health goes downhill." (In other words, you die!)

Even the ancient Greeks knew this. Hippocrates famously said:

"Let food be thy medicine and medicine be

thy food."

And they managed that wisdom without all of our shiny, high-tech gadgets. Imagine that!

What to Eat (And What to Ditch)

Let's get one thing straight: food isn't just about calories. It's *biological fuel.* Every single bite you take is either helping or hurting your metabolism, hormones, mental health, and energy levels.

And yet, moms are constantly being fed conflicting (and often ridiculous) messages:

Eat healthy!

(But also, be quick. You don't have time to cook.)

Make home-cooked meals!

(But don't stress. Just grab something easy.)

Don't drink too much caffeine!

(But how else are you supposed to function?)

It's *exhausting*, and frankly, moms are so over it.

So, instead of obsessing over every single gram of carbs or memorizing a laundry list of fad diets, **let's focus on one thing:**

How does food make you feel? Because when you start eating to fuel your body, instead of just to survive, everything changes.

Ditch the Junk That's Wrecking Your Health

As you have probably picked up on, we're not about perfection here. We're about realistic changes that actually make a difference. And the biggest difference? Getting rid of the stuff that's secretly making you feel like crap.

What to Ditch (Or At Least Cut Way Down On)

Ultra-Processed Foods – If it has a shelf life longer than your child's current obsession with dinosaurs, it's probably not great for you. These foods are engineered to be addictive, packed with inflammatory oils, and disrupt hormones like crazy.

Refined Sugar & Artificial Sweeteners – Sugar is basically the toxic ex-boyfriend of the food world. It spikes your energy, crashes your mood, triggers cravings, and contributes to inflammation, anxiety, and hormone imbalances. And artificial sweeteners? Don't even get me started—they mess with gut health, insulin response, and can actually increase sugar cravings.

Vegetable & Seed Oils (Canola, Soybean, Corn, Sunflower, Safflower, Cottonseed) – These oils are straight-up inflammatory, mess with your metabolism, and contribute to hormone issues. They're in everything from salad dressings to granola bars, so read. your. labels.

Soda & Sugary Drinks – Liquid sugar is a fast track to insulin resistance, weight gain, and energy crashes. Even diet soda isn't safe—it confuses your body, spikes cravings, and messes with gut bacteria.

Refined Carbs (White Bread, Pastries, Most Cereals, Pasta, Crackers) – These spike blood sugar, lead to energy crashes, and contribute to brain fog. If it's made from bleached flour, it's probably not doing you any favors.

Eat More of the Stuff That Actually Nourishes You

Moms don't need to be perfect eaters, we just need to eat food that supports our energy, hormones, and sanity.

Foods That Actually Serve Your Body

Protein, Protein, Protein! – If there's one thing every mom needs more of, it's protein. It stabilizes blood sugar, fuels metabolism, builds muscle (which gives you more energy and fat-burning), and keeps cravings under control.

> **Best sources:** Grass-fed beef, pastured eggs, wild-caught salmon, chicken, turkey, bone broth, Greek yogurt, cottage cheese, and plant-based options like lentils, chickpeas, and hemp seeds.

Healthy Fats – Fats are not the enemy. In fact, good fats are essential for hormone health, brain function, and energy. Plus, they keep you full longer and help prevent sugar cravings.

> **Best sources**: Avocados, olive oil, coconut oil, ghee, grass-fed butter, nuts, seeds, wild-caught fish, and pasture-raised eggs.

Colorful Veggies & Low-Glycemic Fruits – Your gut, hormones, and metabolism *thrive* when you're eating the rainbow. Antioxidants, fiber, and micronutrients are game-changers for digestion, skin, and brain health.

> **Best sources**: Leafy greens, cruciferous veggies (broccoli, cauliflower, Brussels sprouts), bell peppers, zucchini, berries, citrus fruits, and fermented foods (sauerkraut, kimchi, kefir).

Smart Carbs (Because Carbs Are Not All Evil!) – The key is quality. Stick with whole, nutrient-dense carbs that don't spike blood sugar like their ultra-processed cousins.

> **Best sources**: Sweet potatoes, quinoa, lentils, black beans, wild rice, oats, and properly prepared sourdough bread.

Fermented & Gut-Loving Foods – Your gut health controls *everything*. From mood to immunity to digestion. The happier your gut, the better you feel.

> **Best sources**: Greek yogurt, cultured coconut yogurt, sauerkraut, kimchi, kefir, bone broth, and prebiotic foods like garlic, onions, and asparagus.

Hydration is Non-Negotiable – If you're exhausted all the time, you might just be dehydrated. Moms need more liquids than they think—especially if you're drinking caffeine (which is the opposite of hydrating).

Hydration Hacks: Add a pinch of sea salt + lemon to your water, sip on coconut water for electrolytes, and invest in a giant reusable water bottle you actually like using.

And since I know you're short on time, I've included detailed food lists in the Appendix section of the book.

Simplify and Make It Work for Real Life

The goal here isn't to turn you into a Michelin-starred chef. It's to make simple, healthy eating actually doable.

Here's how:

Batch Cook & Meal Prep in a Low-Stress Way – Cook once, eat multiple times. Roast a tray of veggies, cook a big batch of protein, and have grab-and-go options ready (boiled eggs, pre-washed greens, chopped fruit).

Keep Healthy Snacks on Hand – When hunger strikes, having easy options prevents bad decisions. Think nuts, cheese sticks, hard-boiled eggs, hummus and veggies, or protein bars with clean ingredients.

Have a Go-To "Mom Meal" for Chaos Days – Some nights, it's just not happening. Have a backup meal that's nutrient-dense but requires minimal effort (e.g., eggs + avocado toast, a protein smoothie, or a quick stir-fry with frozen veggies).

Swap, Don't Restrict – Instead of cutting things out completely, swap them for better versions:

INSTEAD OF THIS...	TRY THIS...	WHY IT WORKS
White bread	Sprouted grain or sourdough bread	More nutrients, better digestion, fewer blood sugar spikes
Sugary breakfast cereal	Greek yogurt + berries + nuts	More protein, better digestion, longer-lasting energy
Potato chips	Air-popped popcorn w/ sea salt or nuts	Less processed junk, more fiber, and healthy fats
Soda	Sparkling water with lemon or flavored electrolytes	Hydration + no sugar crash
Store-bought salad dressing	Olive oil, balsamic vinegar, and herbs	No seed oils or mystery ingredients

INSTEAD OF THIS...	TRY THIS...	WHY IT WORKS
Fast food burger & fries	Homemade grass-fed burger + roasted sweet potatoes	Better protein + nutrient-rich carbs
Candy bars	Dark chocolate (70%+) with almonds or coconut	Still satisfies the sweet tooth but with antioxidants & healthy fats
Sugary coffee drinks	Black coffee with cinnamon or a homemade latte with nut milk	Less sugar = fewer energy crashes
Canola/corn/soy oil	Extra virgin olive oil, coconut oil, or avocado oil	No inflammation-causing seed oils
White rice	Cauliflower rice, quinoa, or brown rice	More fiber, better blood sugar balance
Milk chocolate	85% dark chocolate or cacao nibs	More antioxidants, less sugar addiction
Ice cream	Frozen banana + nut butter + cacao	Creamy, sweet, and nourishing without the junk
Store-bought granola bars	Homemade energy balls (dates, nuts, coconut, cacao)	No artificial junk, real energy
Sugary flavored yogurt	Full-fat Greek yogurt + raw honey	Less processed sugar, more protein

73

INSTEAD OF THIS...	TRY THIS...	WHY IT WORKS
Fruit juice	Whole fruit with water	Keeps fiber intact, prevents sugar overload
Processed cheese slices	Raw, organic, or goat cheese	Easier to digest, more nutrients
Sugary peanut butter	Natural peanut or almond butter (just nuts & salt)	No added sugar or hydrogenated oils
Packaged protein bars	Hard-boiled eggs or DIY protein balls	More protein, fewer artificial ingredients
White pasta	Chickpea or lentil pasta	More protein & fiber, steadier energy
Store-bought smoothies	Homemade smoothie (greens, berries, protein, nut butter)	No added sugar, actual nutrition
Microwave popcorn	Stovetop popcorn with coconut oil	No toxic chemicals or fake butter
Energy drinks	Matcha or homemade electrolyte drink	No artificial stimulants, more sustained energy
Sugary sports drinks	Coconut water with a pinch of sea salt	Hydration without the sugar dump
Alcohol-heavy nightcap	Herbal tea or kombucha	No hangover, better gut health

Bonus: Mom-Specific Swaps

Instead of starving yourself to "lose the baby weight": *Eat high-protein meals & healthy fats to fuel your day*

Instead of late-night snacking on chips: *Have a protein-rich snack like cottage cheese or nuts to avoid nighttime cravings*

Instead of coffee all day: *Hydrate first with electrolytes to prevent the afternoon crash*

Instead of diet soda: *Try mineral water with lemon & mint for hydration + refreshment*

Instead of skipping meals: *Meal prep easy snacks like boiled eggs, cut-up veggies, & hummus for quick energy*

This chart makes it ***easy to make small, sustainable changes***. No extreme diets, no unrealistic expectations. Just better fuel for a better you!

CHAPTER 09

How Moms Differ

Moms Are Unique-And Overlooked

Trying to balance the demands of family and work or school, and also cope with media pressure to look and eat a certain way, can make it difficult for any woman to maintain a healthy diet. But the right food can not only improve your mood, boost your energy, and help you maintain a healthy weight, it can also support you through the different stages in a mom's life.

As mommas, many of us are frequently prone to neglecting our own dietary needs. You may feel that you're too busy to eat well, or used to putting the needs of your family before your own. Or perhaps you're trying to stick to an extreme diet that leaves you short on vital nutrients and feeling cranky, hungry, and low on energy.

Women's specific needs are often neglected by dietary research too. Nutritional studies tend to rely on male subjects whose hormone levels are more stable and predictable, thus sometimes making the results irrelevant or even misleading to women's needs. For instance, men have a 24 hour cycle of hormone fluctuation versus a woman having a 28 to 32 day cycle of fluctuation-quite a difference, so how can eating the same all day, every day, work for both? It doesn't, plain and simple. This oversight leaves many moms deficient in key vitamins and minerals.

> "The making of hormones requires certain ingredients…I call them the Key 24…We need to eat a variety of nutrient-rich foods to ensure our bodies get all 24 nutrients. When we consume a highly processed, refined food diet, not only is it void of these 24, but these toxic foods also pull nutrients out of our bodies." - Dr. Mindy Pelz, *Fast Like A Girl*

As children, boys' and girls' dietary needs are largely similar. But when puberty begins, women start to develop unique nutritional requirements. And as we age and our bodies go through more physical and hormonal changes, our nutritional needs continue to evolve, making it important that our diets evolve to meet these changing needs.

While moms tend to need fewer calories than dads, our requirements for certain vitamins and minerals are much higher. Hormonal changes associated with menstruation, child-bearing, and menopause mean that women have a higher risk of anemia, weakened bones, and osteoporosis, requiring a higher intake of nutrients such as iron, calcium, magnesium, vitamin D, and vitamin B9 (folate).

Essential Nutrients for Moms:

Here are the **non-negotiables** for women's health:

CALCIUM (1,000-1,200 MG/DAY)

Vital for bone health & mood. (Leafy greens, sardines, tahini, dairy if tolerated.)

MAGNESIUM (320-400 MG/DAY)

Regulates stress & supports sleep. (leafy green vegetables, summer squash, broccoli, halibut, cucumber, green beans, celery, and a variety of seeds.)

VITAMIN D (600 IU/DAY OR PER LAB LEVELS)

Essential for immune function & hormone balance. (half an hour of direct sunlight, and from foods such as salmon, shrimp, vitamin-D fortified milk, cod, and eggs.)

IRON (ADOLESCENT WOMEN AGED 14-18: 15 MG, PREGNANT WOMEN: 27 MG, LACTATING WOMEN 10 MG, ADULT WOMEN 19-50: 18 MG, WOMEN 51+ YEARS OLD: 8 MG)

Prevents fatigue & anemia. (poultry, seafood, dried fruit such as raisins tofu, quinoa, spinach, dark chocolate, nuts and seeds, sweet potatoes, legumes, and apricots,-also cooking in cast iron.)

FOLATE (400-600 MCG/DAY)

Crucial for hormone regulation & cell repair. (Leafy Greens, Legumes, Citrus Fruits, Avocado, Asparagus, Nuts and Seeds, Beets, Broccoli, Brussel Sprouts, Papaya, and Bananas.)

The 411 On Supplements-And Why Vitamins Are Crucial For Women's Health

In the past, women have often tried to make up deficits in their diet through the use of vitamins and supplements. But in some countries, such as the United States, **dietary supplements** are not regulated. It is pretty rare to find a conventional doctor that will run a vitamin deficiency, or nutrient test, to check the levels present in your body. So how on earth would you know if you actually NEED a supplement in the first place? On top of that, the regulations for supplements are just as non-existent as pharmaceuticals. You may be spending your money on a supplement that has less than .5% of the nutrient you are hoping to increase, or none of that nutrient at all. Supplements could also be laced with ingredients that are not even listed on the label. To make sure a supplement is safe and provides the intended nutrients in the stated amounts, look for the symbols *USP (United States Pharmacopeia) or GMP (Good Manufacturing Practices).* Otherwise, you could just be producing very expensive urine.

Furthermore, while verified supplements may be a useful safeguard against occasional nutrient shortfalls, they can't compensate for an unbalanced or unhealthy diet. To ensure you get all the nutrients you need from the food you eat, try to aim for a diet rich in fruit, vegetables, quality protein, **healthy fats,** and stay away from processed, fried, and **sugary food**s.

Time to shift our focus from calorie counting and restrictive diets to nourishing ourselves with positive nutrients (whole foods) and cutting down on negative nutrients (ultra-processed foods). You don't have to be perfect or give up your favorite treats. Just get creative and prioritize nutrient-rich foods to keep your body running smoothly.

Can the food we eat lead to disease?

Our government somehow thinks we are this all powerful nation, but let me set the record straight. The United States ranks ninth in life expectancy among nations in the developed world, and **78 percent of healthcare expenditures are for the treatment of chronic disease** (Anderson and Horvath). I don't know about you, but to me, being powerful means having ultimate strength and control. Spending almost all our healthcare expenditures for all "treatment" required to lift up a sickly nation, doesn't really give off the "strong and in control" vibe.

Finally researchers have come out from hiding to say that these problems are related to diet. (Wow-big applause!) It honestly blows my mind that the citizens of this country have been the ones leading the charge, while our own leaders in government and science are just sitting back, watching (or creating the problems themselves). As Vani Hari (**@thefoodbabe**), a health warrior I deeply respect, put it, "These multinational companies are experts at selling us fake food, produced in massive factories using a laundry list of already processed ingredients. They sell us this junk because it's insanely profitable, even if it means we're consuming a cocktail of dangerous chemicals, additives, and toxic ingredients." She, like so many of us (myself included), has been on the frontlines for years, waving a giant foam finger in their face, but getting through to them is like trying to have a deep conversation with a teenager—good luck with that.

Even my friend Jesse Itzler has tried to push these corrupt companies for accountability, offering the Kellogg's CEO $100,000 to the charity of their choice—just for an interview about the ingredients in their products. And what did he get in return? Nothing. Just crickets. It's tough to change your mind when lobbyists are handing you piles of cash—even if it means people are getting sicker by the day.

While "the royal they" used to believe that diseases - such as type II diabetes, obesity, heart disease, stroke, and certain cancers - were caused by a single gene mutation, they are now generally blaming these conditions on a network of biological dysfunction. Basically our bodies are reacting in defense mode to what we put in it and on it. And the food we eat is a huge factor in that dysfunction, in part because: *our diets suck*. If those statements don't wake you up, our kids are battling the biggest attack of our societal "norm" of diagnosis. Various studies are finding **54% of children in America are diagnosed with chronic illness**. (Yes, you read that correctly.) These numbers continuously climb every year, and they won't stop until we do something about it.

Let's look at autism for example.

In 2001: 1 in 250 kids were diagnosed with Autism

In 2018: 1 in 30 kids were diagnosed with autism (and we know that number is higher in California)

If we continue on this path, by 2028: 1 in 7 will be diagnosed with Autism.

And that's just Autism. We haven't even mentioned asthma, obesity, and mental health disorders. These statistics should piss us off as parents, and wake us up!

Need a real life story to connect the dots of how food impacts the body? Just check out the movie **Super Size Me**. In the film, director Morgan Spurlock documents the negative health outcomes he experienced from eating nothing but fast food for several weeks. It actually grossed me out to the point it was hard to watch. At the end of the experiment, Spurlock had gained 24.5 pounds, a 13% body mass increase, increased his cholesterol, and battled with mood swings, sexual dysfunction, and fat build up in his liver.

Of course, this movie is an extreme example of how food can derail and destroy the balance of health in your body. However, as much as I hate to say it, what was once an out of the ordinary example of eating fast food for every meal is becoming a "normal" program for many families. Even eating just one fast food meal a week can reprogram your body in a negative way.

CHAPTER 10

Food is Medicine
(Or Poison, Your Choice)

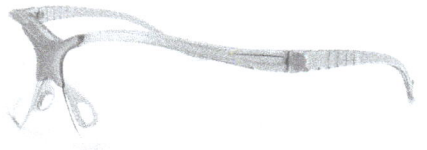

You don't need to count every calorie or stress over every bite. You just need to fuel your body like it actually matters, because it *does*.

► Eat real food: nutrient-dense, unprocessed, and full of healthy fats, quality protein, and fiber.

► Cut out the junk that's secretly draining your energy, inflaming your body, and making you feel *like garbage*.

► Hydrate, sleep, and ditch the all-or-nothing mindset. Progress is better than perfection.

You are not too busy to eat well. You are not too far gone to start feeling better. And you *deserve* to have the energy, clarity, and strength to take care of yourself just as much as you take care of everyone else.

DID YOU KNOW?

Processing removes nutrients

Ever wonder why "processed" sounds like a lot of work? It's because it is! But not in a good way. Processing strips away the nutrients, making the food less healthy and often more addictive. Chemicals like MSG can have an intense grasp on our self control when it comes to cravings, and eventually direct us to eating a specific food-which is why companies use it!

Processed foods have additives

Our typical diet is chock-full of processed foods packed with artificial colors, additives, and chemically altered fats and sweeteners. These additives mess with our bodies, causing inflammation, instead of providing the good stuff we need to function properly.

Even "natural" foods have fewer nutrients

Our food isn't as nutrient-dense as it used to be. Depleted soil and industrial farming practices have resulted in fewer nutrients in our produce and animal products. But, it's still better than the processed junk.

We eat less variety

Despite the introduction of 17,000 new food products each year, two-thirds of our calories come from just four crops: corn, soy, wheat, and rice. Surprise, surprise—these are the ones our government subsidizes!

We eat for convenience, not pleasure

We've shifted from eating for enjoyment and health to eating for speed and convenience. Fast food and drive-thrus have taken over, leaving little room for the simple pleasure of a meal shared around the table. Our digestive systems can barely keep up with the speed at which we consume our food!

So, let's reframe our relationship with food. Instead of seeing it as a chore, or a convenience, let's embrace it as the essential and delightful part of life that it is.

NOW TO THE GOOD STUFF

What is the Impact of Veggies & Fruit?

Unless you live under a rock in a desolate area on the planet, then you are aware of all the amazing benefits that veggies and fruits provide for humans. What **has evolved** from studying the impact of fruits and veggies is the new literature making headlines in the last nine to ten years involving the connection of veggies and fruits' impact on a multitude of diseases. There have been numerous studies, including a study recently published in the American Journal of Clinical Nutrition, showing that eating more fruits and vegetables lowers the incidence of even cardiovascular disease, including strokes. **Who knew eating positive nutrients would give such a positive impact?** (Yes, that was sarcasm!)

Why Protein is the MVP of Your Diet

Protein isn't just about bulking up; it's a powerhouse that keeps your body running smoothly. Whether you're getting it from meats, fish, or beans, protein is essential for your health. While we often talk more about fats and carbs, protein should be in the spotlight as the star since it does a lot of heavy lifting. Here's the lowdown:

Blood sugar and insulin regulation: Protein helps keep your blood sugar and insulin levels balanced, which is key to avoiding those energy crashes. Have high markers of A1C and glucose? Try adding in more protein–and obviously remove sugar.

Mood and sleep hormones: It plays a role in producing hormones that regulate your mood and sleep, keeping you feeling your best and well-rested.

Detoxification: During the second phase of liver detox, protein binds to waste molecules and helps escort them out of your body–so you're literally cleaning house.

Skin, cartilage, and bone health: Protein is vital for making connective tissue, keeping your skin, cartilage, and bones strong and healthy.

Muscle building: It's the building block for muscle growth, which is why you often hear about it in the context of fitness.

Wound healing: Protein speeds up the healing process, making sure your body bounces back quickly–this is key for #momofboys.

Adrenal and thyroid support: It aids in the function of your adrenal and thyroid glands, which are crucial for managing stress and metabolism.

Feeling full: Protein helps you stay full longer, preventing those pesky hunger pangs.

So, when you load up on protein, you're not just feeding your muscles–you're giving your entire body the tools it needs to thrive.

What's the deal with whole grains?

Whole grains are like the secret heroes of your diet, quietly working behind the scenes to keep your body in tip-top shape. Here's why they deserve some love (but don't go overboard):

Steady blood sugar: Unlike their refined counterparts, whole grains are packed with complex carbs that metabolize slowly, keeping your blood sugar levels in check.

Digestive aid: Whole grains help produce good bacteria in your gut, which means better digestion and a happier belly.

Appetite control: The fiber in whole grains tells your brain, "Hey, we're full here!" Helping you avoid overeating.

Cholesterol busters: These grains also play a role in reducing cholesterol, keeping your heart healthy.

Toxin eliminators: Fiber in whole grains binds to toxins in the gut and helps flush them out during elimination. Bye-bye, bad stuff!

Digestive boost: Whole grains improve your digestive system's overall function, making everything run more smoothly.

Neurotransmitter support: They even help synthesize neurotransmitters like serotonin, which is crucial for sleep and mood regulation.

So, next time you are in the mood for some carbs, make it whole grain like quinoa or farrow. But keep it minimal in your daily nutrition-like no more than 1/2 cup uncooked per day. You get more bang for your health buck in heavy carb veggies like sweet potatoes and cauliflower.

Why Fats and Oils Are Your Body's Best Friend (Seriously!)

For years, we've been led to believe that fat is the enemy, thanks to the popularity of low-fat diets. But here's the truth: your body actually *needs* fat to stay healthy. As science catches up, the consensus is shifting—eating the right kinds of fats is crucial for your well-being and disease prevention. Here's why:

Organ insulation: Fats act as a protective cushion for your organs, keeping them safe and secure.

Vitamin transport: They help transport fat-soluble vitamins (A, D, E, K) throughout your body, ensuring you get the most out of these essential nutrients. This is where the term "fat soluble" gets inserted.

Cellular health: Fats are key players in maintaining the integrity of your cell membranes, which keeps everything functioning as it should.

Skin and mucous membrane lubrication: Healthy fats keep your skin and mucous membranes hydrated and happy.

Hormone production: Fats are used by your body to create hormones, which regulate everything from mood to metabolism. Super crucial as we get to perimenopause and menopause.

Glucose utilization: They help your body use glucose more effectively, providing steady energy instead of spikes and crashes.

Joint health: Fats contribute to healthy, well-lubricated joints, making sure you can move freely and without pain.

Gut health: Good fats are essential for maintaining a healthy digestive system, which in turn supports your overall health.

Immune system support: Fats play a role in boosting your immune system, helping you fight off illnesses.

Inflammation control: Depending on the type, fats can either increase or decrease inflammation. Ideally, you want to load up on fats that decrease inflammation, like those from plant oils, nuts, seeds, and fish that thrive on an algae-based diet (hello, omega-3s!).

So, next time you're feeling guilty about eating fat, remember, it's not about avoiding fat; it's about choosing the right ones to keep your body thriving.

How Nutrition Impacts Overall Health & Transitions into Movement

Your diet isn't just about your weight. It impacts every single function of your body, including energy levels, mental clarity, immune function, and even how well your body recovers from daily stress.

Why Your Diet Matters Beyond the Scale

1. **Diet and Cancer:** Your diet influences 30 to 40 percent of all cancers (**BreastCancer.org**) While food alone won't cure or prevent cancer, making smarter choices lowers risk. Focus on antioxidant-rich foods (deep-colored veggies, whole seeds, and nuts) for daily protection.

2. **Protein Power:** Skipping protein = disaster. Your body relies on protein to build muscle, repair tissue, create hormones, and regulate immune function. It's also what

keeps you from collapsing mid-tantrum negotiation and helps you carry the 50-pound car seat without breaking a sweat.

3. **Vitamin and Mineral Magic:** Vitamins and minerals are essential for bone strength, metabolism, and brain function. Vitamin A keeps your skin, bones, and teeth healthy, B vitamins fuel your metabolism, and Vitamin D deficiency can lead to osteoporosis and weakened immunity.

4. **Salt and Blood Pressure:** Instead of fearing salt, embrace the right kind–Redmond's Real Salt, Himalayan pink salt, or sea salt provide essential trace minerals and support thyroid function.

5. **Fiber and Weight Loss:** Fiber helps you stay full longer, stabilizes blood sugar, and prevents overeating. It also supports gut health, aids digestion, and boosts immunity.

6. **Cholesterol & Fiber:** Fiber binds to cholesterol, removing excess from your system before it enters your bloodstream. It's like a bouncer for your arteries–only the good stuff gets through.

7. **Carbs, Blood Sugar, and Weight Gain:** Processed carbs spike your blood sugar and insulin, leading to fat storage, cravings, and energy crashes. Stick to slow-digesting carbs like sweet potatoes, quinoa, and fiber-rich veggies instead.

8. **The Skinny on Fats:** Healthy fats = brain fuel. They help hormone production, nerve function, and cell repair. Stick to olive oil, avocado oil, grass-fed butter, and nuts–not the processed junk.

9. **Sugary Drinks & Disease:** Sugary beverages are directly linked to obesity, diabetes, heart disease, and metabolic dysfunction (**Harvard School of Public Health**). Swap soda for flavored amino acids, sparkling water, or herbal tea.

Nutrition & Mental Health: The Gut-Brain Connection

Your gut is home to billions of bacteria that produce chemicals like dopamine and serotonin: the feel-good neurotransmitters. If your gut is balanced, your brain functions optimally.

- ▶ Eat real food and you will have balanced brain chemistry.
- ▶ Eat sugar and ultra-processed foods and you will have inflammation, mood swings, and anxiety.

Sugar: The Legal Narcotic

- ▶ Sugar triggers the same dopamine surge as drugs like cocaine.
- ▶ It feeds bad gut bacteria, leading to brain fog, anxiety, and energy crashes.
- ▶ More sugar leads to more cravings, which leads to metabolic dysfunction.

When you stick to a diet full of nutrient-dense foods, you're fueling your brain, stabilizing mood, and protecting cognitive function. **Studies** show that clean eating reduces depression and anxiety, while processed diets increase the risk of neurodegenerative diseases.

CHAPTER 11

Stagnant Lifestyle = Stagnant Life

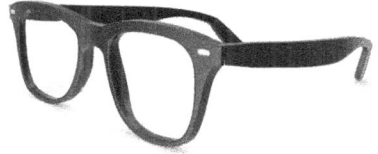

Now that you're fueled with the right nutrition, let's talk about how movement amplifies all these benefits. Exercise isn't just about weight loss, it's about longevity, energy, and stress management.

We've all heard the saying *"sitting is the new smoking"*, right? At first, it might sound like another scare tactic from the health police, but spoiler alert: it's not. The reality is that physical activity takes a nosedive when you become a mom. It's not like you're actively choosing to be sedentary; life just happens. Diaper changes, meal prep, wiping tiny faces, and maybe sneaking in a moment to breathe. **But the numbers don't lie.** Moms today are a third less active than our mothers and grandmothers were. In the '60s, moms were getting about 12.5 hours more of physical activity each week than we are now, and we've added an extra 7 hours of sitting to our daily routines.

If you're thinking, *"But I chase my toddler around all day, isn't that enough?"* Sadly, nope. Moms with younger kids, **especially under five,** see the biggest drop in activity. Stay-at-home moms are hit the hardest, logging more sedentary time than working moms. Up to **75% of moms** experience barriers to regular physical activity, including lack of time and social support, fatigue, childcare, and obligations to other roles, and these barriers were only exacerbated during the COVID-19 pandemic.

And technology isn't helping. Screens have made it easier than ever to binge-watch shows, scroll through social media, and answer emails from anywhere (including bed).

But this isn't just about us feeling tired and sluggish. Our inactivity has a direct effect on our health, and it affects our kids too. **Research shows** that the more active we are, the more active our kids will be. In fact, moms influence their children's exercise habits even more than dads do. For every minute of moderate-to-vigorous activity we do, our kids are more likely to join in with 10% more of their own movement. That means if we can peel ourselves off the couch for an hour, our kids could be less sedentary by at least 10 minutes a day.

Look, I know it's hard. There are so many barriers–lack of time, energy, and let's not even talk about finding childcare so you can squeeze in a workout. But if we want to stop feeling like life is dragging us through the mud, and take back control of our health, we need to get moving–even if it's just a few minutes a day. Baby steps (literally).

What the Heck Is Considered "Stagnant" or "Sedentary", Anyway?

So, what does it really mean to be "stagnant" or "sedentary"? Basically, if your day involves a lot of sitting, reclining, or lying down while barely using any energy, congrats—you've hit the sedentary jackpot. According to a **2017 paper** by the Sedentary Behavior Research Network (SBRN), anything that uses up 1.5 METs (metabolic equivalents) or less is considered sedentary. In non-scientific terms: if you're binge-watching Netflix or scrolling Instagram in bed, that's what we're talking about here.

But here's the thing—just because you're not marathon-training doesn't mean you're doomed. **The U.S. Department of Health and Human Services** suggests that for peak health benefits, you need 150 to 300 minutes of moderate-intensity aerobic activity a week. Sounds intimidating, right? But it doesn't have to be. It's as simple as a brisk 30-minute walk around your block five days a week. Toss in a couple of push-ups or planks before bed, and bam, you're good to go. If you're sitting there thinking, "But who has the time?", well, you're not alone. In fact, a quarter of U.S. adults aren't active at all. And with remote work taking over, the temptation to flop from the computer to the couch to your phone is stronger than ever. I get it. The burnout is real. But here's the deal, we've got to move, not just for us, but so we can actually keep up with our little ones. And if you're able to find a class at a local gym, that's a bonus by meeting other moms that you can work out with.

How a Sedentary Lifestyle Messes with Your Body

Humans were made to move. We're designed to stand upright, walk, lift, and stretch. But modern life has made sitting the default, and it's taking a serious toll. When we're sedentary, we lose energy, our bones weaken, our metabolism slows, and our brains become foggy. Here's what happens when we stop moving:

- ▶ **Legs and Glutes Get Weak:** Sitting all day weakens your leg and glute muscles, making you more prone to injuries.

- ▶ **Weight Gain and Metabolism Slowdown:** Your body needs movement to digest fats and sugars properly. Too much sitting causes fat storage.

- ▶ **Hips and Back Pain:** Sitting for hours tightens hip flexors and weakens back muscles, leading to chronic pain.

- ▶ **Increased Risk of Cancer:** Sitting too much has been linked to lung, uterine, and colon cancers.

- ▶ **Higher Risk of Heart Disease:** Studies show that people who sit for long periods have a 147% higher risk of heart attacks and strokes.

- ▶ **Diabetes Risk Increases:** Just five days of inactivity can spike insulin resistance, putting you at a 112% higher risk of developing diabetes.

- ▶ **Varicose Veins and Blood Clots:** Blood pools in your legs, increasing the risk of blood clots and circulation issues.

So, let's shake off the stiffness, the fatigue, and that third helping of sitting—it's time to get moving!

How to Sneak in More Movement (Without a Gym Membership)

The good news? You don't need a gym, fancy equipment, or hours of free time to get moving. Small changes add up, and every bit of movement counts.

Easy Ways to Add Movement to Your Day:

► Take the stairs instead of the elevator.

► Do squats while brushing your teeth.

► Walk around while taking phone calls.

► Set a timer to get up every hour.

► Turn chores into exercise—vacuuming, mopping, and yard work count!

► Have a 5-minute dance break with the kids (seriously, they'll love it).

► Park farther from the store to sneak in extra steps.

► Stretch before bed to unwind and improve sleep.

Science says you need about 60–75 minutes of moderate activity per day to undo the damage of all that sitting. But don't panic—this doesn't have to happen all at once. A 10-minute walk here, 5 minutes of stretching there—it all adds up.

Simple At-Home Workouts (No Equipment Needed)

10-MINUTE FULL-BODY WORKOUT:

- ► 20 air squats
- ► 15 push-ups (on knees if needed)
- ► 30-second plank
- ► 15 lunges (each leg)
- ► 20 jumping jacks

Repeat 2-3x, or just do what you can!

WALKING & DAILY MOVEMENT GOALS:

- ► Aim for 8,000-10,000 steps per day.
- ► Walk outside daily for sunlight and stress relief.
- ► Try hiking, swimming, biking, or yoga when possible.

YOGA: AN EASY WAY TO GET MOVING

Yoga is one of the best ways to improve flexibility, reduce stress, and build strength, and it's super accessible for moms.

- ► **Hatha Yoga**: Slow and steady–great for beginners.
- ► **Vinyasa Yoga**: More movement, perfect for burning energy.
- ► **Restorative Yoga**: Deep relaxation, perfect before bed.
- ► **Kundalini Yoga**: Uses breathwork and movement for mental clarity.

Even 5-10 minutes of yoga per day can help reduce stress, increase flexibility, and improve mood.

The Impact of a Sedentary Lifestyle on Your Mental Health

Sitting on your butt all day isn't just wrecking your body—it's messing with your mind, too. Yep, the mental toll of a sedentary lifestyle is just as scary as the physical one. **Studies** (Sanchez-Vallegas et al.) have shown that sitting around all day, combined with a lack of physical activity, cranks up your chances of developing a **mental health** disorder. In fact, **recent research** (Zhai et al.) has found a strong connection between sitting too much and an increased risk of **depression**. So, not only is your body paying the price, but your brain's waving the white flag, too.

Anxiety and depression? They love a good sedentary lifestyle. Turns out, spending endless hours lounging can seriously affect your mental state. Less movement means less regulation of blood sugar (hello, mood swings) and leaves you wide open for **cognitive decline**. But here's the good news–researchers found that just 30 minutes of exercise, three to five days a week, can make a real difference in **knocking down those depression and anxiety symptoms**. Thirty minutes! That's like a walk around Target… if you can resist all the distractions.

Thanks to technology, we've pretty much mastered the art of sitting. Whether we're glued to Netflix, doom-scrolling on Social Media, or working from home, we're clocking more screen time than ever. A whopping **80% of adults** spend at least 3 hours a day in front of screens outside of work—that's up from 53% just a decade ago. And guess what? Women are leading the charge. Yay, us?

But it's not just about burning calories or getting steps in. Sitting in front of screens for hours on end messes with the brain chemicals that keep us happy—serotonin and dopamine. Less of those happy hormones means more stress, anxiety, and worse sleep. And let's be real, sleep is already a rare unicorn in mom's life.

On top of all that, being glued to a screen or desk means we're more isolated. We've got fewer chances to interact with people, and those social connections are what keep us sane. Without them, loneliness creeps in, which can trigger all kinds of mental health issues. It's a vicious cycle–sit more, feel worse, repeat.

A study by the **NIH** found that, compared to pre-pandemic times, 39% of moms reported doing less physical activity and 63% were more sedentary. That's not just "mom fatigue"—it's a real problem. And guess what? Nearly a third of moms were dealing with moderate to severe anxiety and depression, and a staggering 78% felt medium to high levels of stress.

I KNOW YOU'RE BUSY AS F*CK, SO HERE'S YOUR CHEAT CODE

Being a mom is no joke. Between wrangling the kiddos and keeping up with your own sanity, squeezing in time for your health feels damn near impossible. But here's the thing—prioritizing your well-being will actually give you more energy to keep up with the chaos. Small, doable changes are where it's at. Let's dive into some easy wins.

Movement Over Exercise

Forget the gym. Just move your body. Getting exercise doesn't have to mean squeezing into spandex and hitting a treadmill for an hour. Push the stroller around the block, park further from the store, chase the kids in the yard. Movement is exercise. The point is, keep moving.

Stock Healthy Snacks

Arm yourself against the 3 p.m. hanger with snacks that won't send your blood sugar into a tailspin. Think almonds, popcorn, string cheese, fruit smoothies, whole fruit. Stock up in your car-you know, the afternoon office that doesn't seem to have a clock out time? They'll keep you fueled without the crash.

Bring the Kids Into Your Workout

Got little ones? Let them join in! Sure, it might slow things down, but running or walking with the stroller still counts. Have them count your reps, or better yet, turn it into a game. Everyone's moving, everyone's happy, and bonus, you're keeping an eye on them while sneaking in some sweat.

Get Creative With Movement

Housework is a workout. Scrubbing floors? You're burning calories. Vacuuming? Same. A 150-pound person can burn about 170 calories an hour doing light chores, and up to 200 calories with tougher tasks. So next time you're mopping, think of it as multitasking: cleaning house and getting fit.

Stay Hydrated, Momma

Water, water, and more water. Hydration keeps you going and helps you avoid those afternoon crashes. Keep a bottle with you and sip on it throughout the day. I'm a big fan of bottles with time markers. They're a solid reminder to keep guzzling.

Plan Ahead (As Best As You Can)

I know, I know, planning with kids is like herding cats. But if you can, jot down a rough schedule the night before. Carve out time for a quick walk, a healthy meal, or even a nap (hey, we can dream!). Having a loose plan helps you squeeze in those healthy habits without feeling like you're scrambling.

Breathe

No joke, sometimes the hardest part of the day is just breathing. When things get chaotic (as they do), take a minute to just stop and breathe. Close your eyes, take three deep breaths, and reset. It sounds simple, but trust me, it works wonders when you're running on fumes.

Find What You Love

Who said working out has to be boring? If you hate running, don't do it. If yoga's not your jam, move on. Find something you enjoy, whether it's dancing, kickboxing, or lifting weights. Mix it up to keep things fun and avoid burnout.

Reduce Stress With Meditation

Parenting is a whole lotta stress. But taking just a few minutes to meditate, read, or simply sit in silence (remember silence?) can seriously help you keep your cool. Try it first thing in the morning or right after the kids crash for the night. Your brain will thank you.

Invest in Simple Home Equipment

Can't make it to the gym? No problem. Invest in a few key pieces of home equipment. Think yoga mat, a couple of dumbbells, or TRX straps. You can get in a solid workout during nap time without ever leaving the house.

Don't Be Afraid to Ask for Help
Finally, don't try to be a supermom all the time. Some days, you just can't do it all, and that's okay. Ask for help. Whether it's your partner, a babysitter, or a friend, give yourself the gift of a few hours to recharge. It's not weakness, it's survival.

Move More, Feel Better
Moms are busier than ever, and fitting in exercise might feel like an impossible task. Movement isn't just for weight loss. It's for energy, mental clarity, stress relief, and long-term health.

Start small. Take the stairs. Walk outside. Stretch before bed. Every little bit counts. You don't need a perfect workout routine—just movement.

You're not just moving for yourself, you're setting the example for your kids. They learn from watching you. Show them that taking care of your body matters.

Let go of the guilt. Embrace the chaos. Just move. You've got this.

CHAPTER 12

Sleep–The Foundation of Everything

Now that we have nutrition and movement down (well, at least we've discussed it, and we know the effort will begin soon), let's chat about sleep. Remember that thing you used to do before kids?

Between feeding schedules, school runs, work stress, and general chaos, restful sleep feels like a distant fantasy. But just because you're a mom doesn't mean you have to settle for a life of constant exhaustion. Prioritizing good sleep might just be the most important thing you do for your sanity, health, and family.

Now, let's not forget how the medical industry and society have totally screwed up sleep hygiene over the years. From pushing quick-fix sleep aids to glorifying the "tired mom" as a badge of honor, it's no wonder moms everywhere are walking around like zombies. Let's break down how we got here, why sleep is crucial (duh), and how you can reclaim it *without* relying on a pill.

How the Medical Industry & Society Messed with Your Sleep

Let's talk about how things have gone wrong. Over the last few decades, the pharmaceutical industry has made bank off sleep-deprived moms, pushing prescription sleep aids like Ambien, Lunesta, and others as the magic cure for insomnia. They've marketed these drugs with pictures of well-rested women, ignoring the fact that these pills often come with a laundry list of side effects. Including dependence, grogginess, and impaired functioning-which kinda throws a wrench in the afternoon taxi driving.

These sleep aids are a multi-billion-dollar industry, but they don't fix the root cause of your sleeplessness. Instead, they put a band-aid on the issue while the real problems (stress, hormone imbalances, lack of proper sleep hygiene) go unaddressed. So what do we end up with? Moms who are *technically* sleeping but still waking up feeling like they've been hit by a bus.

The push for pharmaceutical solutions has also loosened regulation over time. Drugs that are supposed to be for short-term use often get prescribed long-term, despite clear warnings. And who's the victim here? Moms, who are trying to juggle it all and end up feeling like they need a pill just to survive. It's not your fault. Our healthcare system has basically programmed us to believe that a quick fix is the only solution.

Then there's society itself, glorifying burnout and exhaustion. We're told we need to "do it all," wearing our lack of sleep like a badge of honor. All of us strive to be the perfect "bot mom", but there's a problem. We're not bots, we're humans. It's no wonder we're running on fumes.

Why Sleep Matters (More Than Ever)

We all know sleep is important, but sleep deprivation messes with everything. Your health, mood, and even your waistline. Research shows that poor sleep increases the risk of heart disease, diabetes, depression, and even early death. Moms are especially vulnerable, since sleep deprivation can turn patience into irritability and make you feel like you're constantly in survival mode.

New studies have shown that consistently getting less than six hours of sleep a night messes with your hormones, wrecks your metabolism, and can even age you faster (yikes). *The Journal of Sleep Research* **recently reported that losing just 16 minutes of sleep a night negatively impacts mood, focus, and emotional resilience.** It's a big deal, especially when you've got little ones depending on you.

But popping a sleeping pill isn't the answer. It might get you through the night, but the next day? You're still groggy and running on fumes.

Why Sleep Matters:

1 **Regulates hormones** (cortisol, leptin, ghrelin—aka stress and hunger hormones)

Why Sleep Matters:

2 Improves mood and reduces anxiety

3 Boosts immune system (less sick days!)

4 Balances blood sugar and prevents weight gain

The Downside of Lack of Sleep

Sleep is like a mythical unicorn we moms are constantly chasing but never quite catching. You're exhausted, but you still can't sleep. Or worse, you finally get to sleep, and someone's tiny voice yells, *"Mommy, I had a bad dream!"* Cue the sleepless nights and coffee-fueled mornings. Let's not sugarcoat it—sleep deprivation is wrecking your health, body, and let's face it, your soul. Here's how this sneaky little thief messes with both your physical and mental well-being:

1. Physical Well-Being:
Sleep Deprivation's Attack Plan
Hormonal Havoc

Forget hormonal balance, lack of sleep throws your system into chaos. Say hello to cortisol spikes, insulin resistance, and *why-does-my-face-look-like-this* mornings. Your body's like, "Cool, let's hoard fat and mess up your metabolism while we're at it."

Immune System Meltdown

You know that cold you can't shake or the never-ending flu season in your house? Thank your sleepless nights. Your immune system goes on strike without proper rest, leaving you open to every germ your kid brings home from daycare.

Accelerated Aging

Bags under your eyes? Check. Dull, tired skin? Double check. Chronic sleep deprivation doesn't just make you feel older; it makes you *look* older too. Talk about unfairness

Increased Risk of Chronic Disease

Heart disease, diabetes, obesity, oh my! Skimping on sleep puts you at risk for the big stuff. Not terrifying at all, right?

Poor Physical Recovery

Sleep is when your body repairs itself, but when you're running on fumes, your body's like, "Nah, we'll just leave those muscles sore and that wound healing slow. Good luck!"

2. Mental Well-Being: The Spiral Into Crazy Town

Mood Swings that Rival a Teenager

Lack of sleep can turn the sweetest mom into a raging lunatic faster than a toddler can smear peanut butter on the couch. One minute you're crying over spilled milk; the next, you're yelling because someone dared to breathe near you.

Memory Lapses & Brain Fog

You walk into a room and forget why you're there. You call your kid the dog's name. Sleep deprivation messes with your brain, making you feel like you're losing it, because you kind of are.

Skyrocketing Anxiety

Did you know that sleep deprivation amps up your stress levels? That endless loop of *"Am I doing enough?"* and *"What did I forget today?"* gets louder when your brain's running on empty.

Decreased Patience

Sleep-deprived moms have the patience of a hangry toddler. Cue the guilt trip when you snap at your kids for asking the same question 300 times.

Increased Risk of Depression

Chronic sleep deprivation can fuel postpartum depression or intensify already-existing mental health struggles. You're not just tired; you're spiraling, and it's a big deal.

Diminished Coping Skills

Little annoyances feel like the apocalypse when you're running on three hours of sleep. No, Karen, I don't want your parenting advice right now.

The Alternative to Pills: Natural Sleep Solutions for Moms

Before you reach for that bottle of Ambien, let's talk about simple, effective ways to improve your sleep naturally. These methods are easy to integrate into your life, don't come with nasty side effects, and, bonus, you won't be dependent on Big Pharma for a good night's rest. I'll go more in depth on each of these in the second part of this book, but here are the cliff's notes version:

1. Create a Sleep-Inducing Environment

Your bedroom needs to be a sanctuary. Think cool, dark, and quiet. Blackout curtains are a mom's best friend, and if you've got a snoring partner or noisy neighbors, a white noise machine can be a lifesaver.

2. Stick to a Sleep Schedule

Your body thrives on routine, even if your toddler doesn't.

Try to go to bed and wake up at the same time every day, even on weekends. This keeps your circadian rhythm in check, helping you fall asleep easier and wake up refreshed.

I know it's tough when you've got kids, but consistency is key. And if you've got a baby or toddler who wakes you up constantly, aim to at least get yourself into a rhythm with naps.

3. Ditch the Caffeine

As tempting as that afternoon cup of coffee is, try swapping it out for something caffeine-free. Caffeine has a sneaky way of sticking around in your system for hours, and it might be sabotaging your ability to sleep later. The worst part? You might not even realize it's affecting you until you're lying in bed wide awake at midnight. Herbal teas like chamomile or peppermint can be a great substitute. They're calming and won't keep you wired all night.

4. Practice Mindfulness Before Bed

Mom brain doesn't have an off switch. That to-do list keeps running, and next thing you know, you're lying awake stressing about everything you didn't get done. Mindfulness and meditation can help you hit pause on the mental chaos and prepare your mind for rest. Even five minutes of deep breathing can work wonders.

5. Natural Sleep Aids

If you need a little extra help falling asleep, consider natural supplements like magnesium, melatonin, or valerian root. Magnesium is great for relaxing your muscles and calming your nervous system, while melatonin gives you that gentle nudge toward dreamland. Valerian root has been used for centuries to help with anxiety and sleep issues. *If you are on medications, always check with your doctor before trying any natural herb out. While these are nature's remedies, they can be extremely potent.

6. Move During the Day

Exercise is a great way to regulate your sleep, but you don't need to spend hours at the gym. A brisk walk, a quick yoga session, or chasing your kids around the park is enough to keep your body in motion and improve your sleep at night.

7. Watch Your Diet

What you eat affects how you sleep. Heavy meals or sugary snacks before bed can mess with your ability to fall asleep and stay asleep. If you're hungry before bed, opt for light, sleep-friendly snacks like a banana, almonds, pistachios, or a small handful of walnuts. Foods that help produce melatonin naturally.

8. Give Yourself Grace

Sleep with kids is unpredictable, plain and simple. Some nights, it just won't happen. That's okay. Give yourself grace and nap when you can. Don't beat yourself up if things don't go according to plan. Tomorrow is another chance to try again.

9. Seed Cycling

A method that doesn't just focus on gobbling down seeds all day long. This is based on alternative and integrative medicine practices. The benefits people see from utilizing this method is a balance of hormones, and assists in a better night's sleep.

10. Shut Off The Screens...No, Seriously!

I felt the need to elaborate on screen usage, especially with the crazy amount of usage in today's world. So, all this screen time: what is it really doing to us?

Spoiler alert: It's not doing us any favors. Sure, our phones, tablets, and laptops keep us connected, entertained, and momentarily sane, but that much screen time? It's taking a toll, especially on our eyes and sleep. And, no, just putting your phone on "night mode" isn't enough.

Easy Nighttime Routine for Better Sleep

1. **Dim lights after sunset** (signals your brain it's time to wind down)

2. **Drink herbal tea** (chamomile, reishi, or valerian root)

3. **Stretch or foam roll** (relaxes your nervous system)

4. **Take magnesium or collagen powder** (supports deep sleep)

5. **Read (not scroll)** to help your brain power down

The Point I Need To Make With Screens

So, what's the deal with blue light? Blue light is part of the visible light spectrum (yep, the stuff our eyes can see) and it's got the shortest wavelength and highest energy. About a third of all visible light is blue light, with the biggest source being. You guessed it, the sun. The issue: we're now getting a hefty dose of it from artificial sources like LED TVs, computer monitors, and every single one of those devices we're glued to all day. And while blue light in moderation has its perks (it boosts alertness, helps brain function, and keeps our circadian rhythm in check), too much of it is where things start going south.

Check out these numbers: **80% of American adults** use digital devices for more than two hours a day, and nearly 67% are juggling two or more screens at once. It's a screen-palooza! And what's the price we pay? Eye strain, headaches, dry eyes, blurred vision, you name it. Since our eyes don't naturally block blue light, almost all of it hits the retina, which over time could lead to some serious vision problems like macular degeneration, cataracts, or even eye cancer. And get this–**kids are even more at risk** because their eyes soak up more blue light than ours.

Scrolling through social media in bed or binge-watching your favorite show before dozing off can mess with your melatonin production, which is your body's natural "get sleepy" hormone. When your melatonin levels are off, it throws your **whole circadian rhythm** out of whack, making it harder to fall asleep or stay asleep.

Now, will blue light glasses save the day? Maybe. There's no unanimous verdict from the science squad, but some studies suggest they might help ease eye strain from all that screen time. They won't cure the problem, but they can give your eyes a little break. Plus, they might help you sleep better if you're staring at screens all day.

But even if you're not into rocking the blue light glasses, there are other ways to save your eyes. Slap a blue-light filter on your devices and follow the 20-20-20 rule: every 20 minutes, look at something 20 feet away for 20 seconds. Your eyes will thank you. Oh, and make sure your screens aren't too bright and that your workspace isn't all shadows and glares. Minor tweaks can make a big difference. So yeah, the screens aren't going any-where, but neither is your eye health (hopefully).

CHAPTER 13

The Perfection Trap

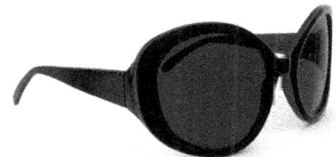

The absurdity of modern motherhood is this: society tells us to "have it all"—the thriving career, the Pinterest-perfect home, the well-behaved kids, the six-pack abs—and to do it all with a smile on our face. No pressure, right?

And just when we think we might be figuring it out, social media swoops in with an endless highlight reel of moms who seem to have it all together. Perfect family vacations, spotless kitchens, well-rested faces (seriously, how?!). Suddenly, what we have feels like it isn't enough. We're not enough.

But here's the truth: comparison is a dirty thief. It steals our joy, our confidence, and our ability to see our own lives clearly. It's time to break the cycle and take back our self-worth.

Societal Blockers: The Social Media Trap

Welcome to the social media jungle, where every mom is a

"bot mom" with perfectly groomed kids, immaculate homes, and effortless parenting.

Social media is packed with these idealized snapshots, and let's be real. It's completely unrealistic and phony. These polished portrayals make us feel like we're constantly falling short. We scroll through our feeds, comparing ourselves to other moms who seem to have it all together, amplifying stress and self-doubt. The pressure to match these idealized standards pulls us further away from the messy reality of parenting, making us hide our struggles, out of fear of judgment.

I've been there. I still battle the Goliath of self-loathing when I compare myself to other moms online. How many times have you been having "a day," thrown your hair into a messy bun, put on sweats, and felt like doing absolutely nothing (only to scroll and see a perfectly put-together mom giving you tips on "the best way to organize your life")? Yup, I've wanted to throw my phone at the wall too.

When we get sucked into comparison mode, it hits our self-esteem hard. Studies show that social comparison (Kirkpatrick and Lee) is linked to higher levels of depression and anxiety, triggering our fight-or-flight response and releasing cortisol and adrenaline, the very hormones we need less of. Over time, this stress takes a major toll on mental and physical health, adding to the already heavy mental load moms carry.

The Push Toward Cosmetic Procedures: Is This Really the Answer?

When the pressure to look perfect gets too loud, the cosmetic industry swoops in with promises of quick fixes. Botox, fillers, implants, and weight loss shots, whatever it takes to look like you just stepped out of a glossy magazine. The message? If you're not perfect, don't worry; there's a procedure for that. Except it's a never-ending cycle of "fixing" and still feeling like you're not enough. We should be grateful to "age with grace" or "wear our scars and stretch marks with pride". Some moms don't get that honor or privilege. We may not look "perfect", but what is "perfect"?

We live in an extremely contradictory society of "you should love yourself for who you are"; but also, "if you don't like how you look, you should absolutely be able to change that and feel confident in who you are". Ummmmm…what?!

Is society encouraging self-love or body dysmorphia? Because it sure feels like both. And trust me, I know this first-hand.

Boob-Free and Fabulous: My Journey Through Body Image & Explant Surgery

For as long as I can remember, I struggled with body dysmorphia.

My boobs were too big. My back hurt. I felt self-conscious in everything I wore.

I thought that surgery would fix it. By the time I was done nursing my kids, I was fully committed to getting a breast reduction. I wanted relief. I wanted to feel lighter. I wanted to love my body.

But when I met with my surgeon, I was told that a breast lift with implants was the "best option." He played on my emotions, convincing me that starting my 30s with non-perky breasts would be a confidence shut down for me. At the time, I was so mortified by how my body looked, I would listen to anyone who was seen as "an expert". There was no conversation about a natural lift, or a fat lipid transfer. No natural methods to give me the "supple" look he wanted me to go for. (It seriously makes me nauseous thinking about the consultation now.)

It made no sense, why add volume when I wanted to reduce? But my surgeon, like so many others, had one goal: to meet society's version of "aesthetically pleasing." His convincing statements sealed my choice. I chose to trust the process.

When the "Fix" Became the Problem

For the first year after surgery, everything seemed great. But then my body started betraying me.

Extreme fatigue—beyond "mom tired."

Brain fog that made it hard to function.

Itchy skin that wouldn't go away.

Blurry vision.

Tingling and numbness in my fingers and toes.

Irregular cycles and sleep disturbances.

I felt like I was falling apart.

Doctors were zero help. I was dismissed with:

"You're just a tired mom."

"Maybe you're stressed."

"Let's try antidepressants."

Finally, after years of struggling, I was diagnosed with Hashimoto's Thyroiditis and Hypothyroidism (along with a long laundry list of gut health issues).

Among all the research I had been doing on integrative health, gut health, and detoxification, I discovered Breast Implant Illness (BII). The timing was too suspicious. The symptoms lined up exactly. My immune system went into overdrive the year after foreign objects were placed in my body.

I had fought for years to "fix" my body. Now, my body was fighting back.

The Realization:
My Body Was Never the Problem

The problem wasn't my boobs. The problem wasn't my body. The problem was the sick and twisted manipulation that I needed to "look" a certain way when I was 30. So I made a new decision—I was getting my implants removed.

Breaking Free from Society's Lies

This time, I chose a surgeon who actually cared about my whole health.

Prepping for surgery wasn't about aesthetics.

I strengthened my body beforehand.

I ate for healing, not weight loss.

I worked on my mental and emotional well-being.

And post-op care wasn't just about resting.

Lymphatic drainage to detox my system.

Hyperbaric oxygen therapy to accelerate healing.

Functional medicine oversight to rebuild my health.

It was a night and day difference.

Healing Through Self-Love

You know what's ironic? For years, I hated my body. I tried to shrink it. I tried to reshape it. I tried to fix what was never broken.

And now? I'm boob-free and fabulous. Not because my body is "perfect."

But because I finally stopped fighting it.

The Impossible Beauty Standards That Trap Moms

We live in a world that preaches self-love but profits off of insecurity. We're told to "love ourselves as we are," but also, "there's a procedure for that flaw if you really need to fix it." Umm… which is it?

It's no surprise that the cosmetic industry is thriving, fueled by the relentless pressure on women to maintain impossible beauty standards. In 2019 alone, women underwent 1.5 million cosmetic surgeries and 13.4 million minimally invasive treatments. What does that tell us? That society is setting us up to feel like we're never enough.

I fell for it too.

But here's the truth:

You don't have to be "fixed."

You don't have to chase an impossible standard.

You don't have to sacrifice your health to "fit in."

Your body is a f*cking miracle.

It carried life. It nurtures and protects. It deserves respect, not toxic implants, injections, or treatments. If you want to make changes, do it for YOU, not for someone else's approval. Because loving yourself isn't about "fixing" your body. It's about choosing yourself, as you are, every single day.

A Closer Look at Popular Cosmetic Procedures

The pressure to achieve the "perfect" body has led many women to seek out cosmetic procedures, but the reality is often far from the flawless results promised. Take breast implants, for example they might seem like an easy way to enhance curves, but they come with serious risks, including implant ruptures, chronic fatigue, joint pain, autoimmune issues, and BII. That "quick fix" can quickly turn into years of complications. A safer, more natural alternative? Strength training and targeted breast-lifting exercises. Bonus: Yoga not only improves posture but also gives both the chest and glutes a natural lift, no surgery required.

Weight loss injections like Semaglutide (Ozempic, Wegovy), Tirzepatide (Mounjaro), Liraglutide (Saxenda), Phentermine, and HCG promise effortless weight loss, but at what cost? Side effects range from nausea and hair loss to thyroid cancer risks, and a metabolism that can end up completely out of whack. Instead of relying on a needle, an anti-inflammatory diet combined with mindful movement (walking, yoga, and strength training) offers sustainable, long-term results without the dangerous side effects.

Then there's Botox and fillers, the go-to for smoothing wrinkles and keeping skin looking youthful. While they might seem harmless, the potential downsides include droopy eyelids, facial asymmetry, and the unsettling fact that fillers don't fully break down in the body. Once they're in, they stay in. A better alternative? Facial yoga and Gua Sha help tone, lift, and improve circulation for a naturally radiant complexion, no injections required.

Prescription diet pills like Adderall and Phentermine are another tempting shortcut, offering quick weight loss, an energy boost, and sharper focus. But these benefits come with a high price—heart palpitations, insomnia, addiction, and long-term heart damage. Instead of putting your health at risk, natural adaptogens like Ashwagandha and Rhodiola provide a safer way to boost energy and manage stress, while a well-balanced diet ensures your body stays fueled the right way.

At the end of the day, the cosmetic and pharmaceutical industries thrive on selling quick fixes, but the trade-offs often outweigh the benefits. Choosing natural alternatives not only protects your health but also supports long-term well-being, without the hidden risks.

THE EMOTIONAL TOLL

Feeling "Not Good Enough" After Cosmetic Procedures

Here's a not-so-fun fact: cosmetic procedures don't magically wave a wand over your self-esteem and make it sparkle. Sure, they might tweak a nose here or smooth a wrinkle there, but they won't fix the deeper belief that you're not good enough. Even worse, the pursuit of perfection can become a never-ending hamster wheel, leaving you more exhausted and disappointed when the results don't live up to your expectations, or when new insecurities pop up out of "nowhere". The truth is, no scalpel or syringe can fill the void created by a society that tells moms they need to "bounce back" or look perfect to be worthy. Guess what: you were already worthy.

The Hidden Mental Health Impacts

Here's the thing: cosmetic surgery might change your reflection in the mirror, but it won't magically heal those deeper self-image issues lurking beneath the surface. In fact, for some, going under the knife can backfire, making feelings of anxiety, depression, or even body dysmorphia worse. It's like slapping a Band-Aid on a bullet wound, it might cover things up for a while, but it doesn't address the real problem. The reality is, true confidence isn't something that can be injected, sculpted, or airbrushed into existence. It's built from within, and no amount of nips or tucks can replace the work it takes to genuinely love and accept yourself, flaws and all.

Reclaiming Your Authentic Beauty: Natural Alternatives to Cosmetic Procedures

Building Confidence from Within

True confidence starts from within, and it's about embracing a mindset that prioritizes health, well-being, and self-acceptance over chasing superficial ideals. Shifting your focus to what truly matters: feeling strong, energized, and comfortable in your skin, can be incredibly empowering. Instead of scrutinizing perceived flaws, celebrate your body for its strength and resilience, especially in the postpartum phase. This incredible vessel has created life, endured sleepless nights, and adapted to countless challenges. Honoring its journey and achievements can help shift the narrative from criticism to gratitude. Confidence doesn't come from conforming to society's impossible standards but from recognizing your worth as you are right now.

Mindset Shift: Health, well-being, and self-acceptance > superficial aesthetics

Body Positivity: Celebrate your postpartum body for its strength and resilience. It created life, after all!

Nutritional Alternatives for Glowing Skin and Hair

Radiant skin and luscious hair don't have to come from a bottle or a procedure, they can start right in your kitchen. By nourishing your body with the right foods, you can eat your way to natural beauty that lasts. Antioxidant-packed foods like vibrant berries and leafy greens work wonders to fight off skin-damaging free radicals, keeping your complexion bright and youthful. Omega-3 fatty acids found in salmon, walnuts, and flaxseeds are like a secret weapon for hydration and elasticity, giving both your skin and hair a healthy glow. And don't forget collagen-boosting nutrients like vitamin C and zinc, which support your skin's structure and repair, ensuring it stays firm and radiant. When you fuel your body with these powerhouse nutrients, you're not just improving your appearance—you're laying the foundation for long-term health and vitality.

Eat Your Way to Radiance: Antioxidant-packed foods (berries, leafy greens), Omega-3s (salmon, flaxseeds), and collagen-boosting nutrients (vitamin C, zinc) will have your skin and hair thriving.

Lifestyle Practices for Natural Beauty

When it comes to natural beauty, lifestyle habits are the unsung heroes. Let's start with sleep—yes, beauty sleep is a real thing! Prioritizing quality rest doesn't just leave you feeling refreshed; it actively reduces stress hormones and promotes cellular repair, giving your skin that coveted glow. Next up is hydration, the ultimate skincare product that costs practically nothing. Drinking plenty of water helps flush out toxins, keeps your skin plump, and maintains that dewy look from the inside out. And let's not forget stress management. Practices like meditation, breathwork, and mindfulness aren't just for your mental health; they also help prevent those pesky stress-induced wrinkles and frown lines. Together, these simple lifestyle habits create a foundation for natural beauty that no cream or procedure can replicate.

Prioritize Sleep: Beauty sleep is real, folks. Rest reduces stress and promotes cell repair.

Hydration: Water is the OG skincare product. Drink up!

Stress Management: Meditation, breathwork, and mindfulness can keep those stress-induced wrinkles at bay.

The Takeaway:
Rejecting False Beauty Standards

It's time to stop the madness and step off the hamster wheel of society's impossible beauty standards. Let's be honest—no one can keep up with the ever-changing expectations of perfection-whatever that is, and trying to do so only drains your energy and happiness. What truly matters is your health, your joy, and your ability to show up fully for yourself and your family. Real empowerment comes from embracing self-care practices that make you feel good from the inside out, not from chasing what others think you should look like.

Empowerment Through Self-Care
Prioritize what makes you feel good inside and out— not what society says you should look like.

The Importance of Setting a Positive Example
Teach your kids that real beauty isn't about flawless skin or a perfect figure. It's about being strong, confident, and unapologetically yourself.

By rejecting these false ideals, you're also sending a powerful message to your children. Teaching them that beauty isn't about flawless skin, a perfect figure, or meeting anyone else's definition is one of the greatest gifts you can give. Instead, show them that true beauty lies in being strong, healthy, confident, and unapologetically yourself. When you prioritize your well-being and embrace who you are, you lead by example, demonstrating that self-worth isn't found in a mirror but in how you live your life. So let go of the pressure, embrace your imperfections, and remind yourself that you are already enough. Because you are.

RECLAIMING YOUR AUTHENTIC BEAUTY

True confidence isn't found in a bottle of filler or a diet pill. It's found in **self-acceptance**.

► **Your body is not a problem to be fixed.**

► **You are not defined by a number on a scale.**

► **Your worth is not tied to your appearance.**

Instead of **chasing perfection, chase self-respect**. Instead of **fixing yourself, start nurturing yourself**. Instead of **comparing, start celebrating**.

Because, Mama? **You are already enough**.

Setting a New Standard

Our daughters and sons are watching. If we want them to grow up knowing their worth isn't tied to their looks, we have to model that truth for them. Let's stop apologizing for our bodies. Let's stop chasing an illusion of perfection. Let's redefine beauty—on our own terms.

It starts with us.

And it starts now.

CHAPTER 14

The Power of Community

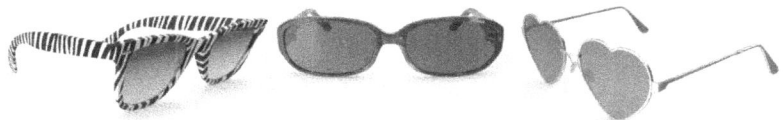

Picture this: you're running around like a wild woman, tackling everything from baby cries to laundry piles, barking dogs to ringing doorbells. By the time you finally sit down and catch a breath, there it is—that wave of emptiness that hits you out of nowhere. It takes a second to name it, but then it clicks: loneliness.

Yeah, that one hits hard.

Motherhood comes with its own little identity crisis, doesn't it?

Your body? Unrecognizable and slightly uncomfortable.

Relationship with your partner? Let's just say... "evolved."

Career? Yep, that changed too.

Priorities? Completely flipped.

Friendships? Wait, where did they go?

The thing is, we're sold this ideal of motherhood as the ultimate time of joy and fulfillment. But that picture-perfect version conveniently forgets the messiness. No one mentions the sleep deprivation, the insane pressure to be a "good" mom, or how isolating it can feel to be up to your elbows in diapers, with only your own thoughts for company. It's no surprise that loneliness among moms is rampant, and it's taking a serious toll on our mental and physical health.

When you bring a tiny human into the world, it shakes everything up. Your relationships, your social life, your job, your values. Everything shifts, and you're left trying to keep it all together with whatever sanity you have left. Despite common societal expectations that it should be the 'happiest time of their life', women are vulnerable to developing psychological distress and mental health problems during the perinatal period. In particular, depression affects approximately **one in six** pregnant women and **one in five** women during the first 3 months after birth.

We've got the stats to prove it, too. **Harvard University** conducted a national survey in 2021, and guess what? A whopping 36% of American adults said they felt lonely frequently. For young people aged 18–25, that number jumps to 61%, and for moms of young kids, it's 51%. A more recent **Motherly** survey in 2024 found that **85% of moms reported feeling lonely or isolated after becoming a parent.**

So, it's official: many of us are feeling lonely. And the best part? We're talking about it now. Because loneliness doesn't win here. We're all navigating this together, even when it feels like we're worlds apart.

Social Isolation vs. Loneliness: The Fine Line Between "Alone" and "Lonely"

Social isolation is that very real, measurable lack of social connection. It's the stuff we can count: limited contact with friends and family, having fewer than a handful of close confidants, or not belonging to any social groups. It's living alone, not having anyone to call for a quick vent session, and feeling like you've been sidelined from the team.

But don't think social isolation just messes with your social calendar—it's as dangerous as smoking 15 cigarettes a day. **Julianne Holt-Lunstad,** a professor of psychology and neuroscience at BYU, even found that social isolation can be twice as harmful to your health as obesity. And it's not just hitting us hard; it's hitting **our kids too**. Kids without social connections have a harder time in school, struggle with mental health, and often face challenges in their development. Without regular social interactions, **they're more likely to feel** socially anxious, have trouble making friends, and could face cognitive and speech delays.

Now, loneliness is a whole different animal. Loneliness is what we feel, not just what we see. It's that empty, disconnected feeling you get even when you're surrounded by people. It's the emotional gap between the kind of social life you want and what you've actually got.

Emotional Impact of Loneliness on Moms

When loneliness moves in, it doesn't just affect how we feel—it messes with our mental health big time.

*A **study** published in 2019 found that moms
who reported feeling lonely were three times*

*more likely to experience symptoms of depression than those who felt connected. And it's a **major player in postpartum depression**, which affects about **one in seven new moms.***

Once loneliness rears its ugly head, it has a way of making you question everything—yourself, your relationships, and your worth as a mom.

And let's not forget anxiety. **In 2020,** research showed that **lonely mothers were two and a half times more likely to experience significant anxiety symptoms.** The worry feels heavier, the "what ifs" never stop, and suddenly, you're spiraling into a cycle that feels impossible to get out of.

Self-Esteem, Identity, and the Constant Struggle

Loneliness doesn't stop at anxiety and depression. It goes straight for your self-esteem. **Research** shows that moms experiencing chronic loneliness often struggle with their sense of identity. It's like trying to reconcile who you were before becoming a mom with who you are now, and loneliness is the nagging voice that keeps telling you you're not measuring up.

Burnout: The Final Straw

Moms have enough on their plate without loneliness creeping in and draining whatever energy is left. A study in **2022** found that lonely mothers were 1.7 times more likely to experience parental burnout, and that's just the emotional side of things. When we're lonely, our bodies feel it. We're wired for connection, and when that connection's missing, our bodies kick into survival mode. Every system feels the strain, from our immune system to our stress levels.

So, whether it's social isolation, loneliness, or both, the effects are real, and they're intense. The good news? You're not alone in feeling alone. And recognizing it is the first step to breaking the cycle.

Why Are Moms So Lonely?

Motherhood can feel like a one-way ticket to Loneliness-ville. Suddenly, your life revolves around someone else's every need 24/7, and things like sleep, "me time," and sanity seem like distant memories. You're expected to manage every hiccup, diaper change, and meltdown without missing a beat, often with little or no support. And while everyone talks about the joy of motherhood, no one really prepares you for just how isolating it can be.

Let's face it: Loneliness is practically a rite of passage in parenthood. Dr. Aparna Iyer, a psychiatrist focused on reproductive mental health, puts it like this: "So much of parenting feels like a solo journey—the late-night feeds, the endless diaper changes, the breastfeeding struggles—that moms often feel lonely even with their partners right beside them." And throw in any mental health challenges, and it can feel even more isolating.

The numbers paint a pretty bleak picture, too. **Studies by Cigna** in 2021 found that 65% of parents are considered lonely, compared to 55% of non-parents. For moms, it's even worse—69% experience loneliness, compared to 62% of dads. Single moms? A staggering 77% report feeling lonely. And honestly, are we surprised? The journey of motherhood is transformative, yes, but it can also leave you feeling like a stranger in your own life.

Here's another thing: you're still you, but now you're also a mom. You might have less in common with friends who don't have kids, and let's be real, they probably don't want to hear about diaper rashes or the latest toddler tantrum. Add to that the constant solo care of an infant or toddler—it's not like you're getting much adult conversation in when you're stuck in a loop of feeds, naps, and diaper changes. Even as your kids get older, your life still revolves around their schedules, their needs, and the daily grind of balancing work, home, and activities. Building and maintaining friendships is tough when you're already stretched so thin. Even planning one lunch outing can feel like you're planning the event of the century–just trying to figure out the day and time that work for both of you.

Then, there's the cultural expectation that "we should do it all with a smile." Multigenerational homes are not the norm, so many of us don't have built-in help, and asking for help? That's practically stigmatized. And our society loves to sell this image that moms should be able to juggle it all, as if asking for help is some sort of parenting failure.

Let's not forget the cherry on top: COVID-19. The pandemic didn't just turn our lives upside down; it magnified the loneliness, especially for moms who lost any social outlets they had. Plus, the constant friction over health and safety measures—everyone had an opinion—added another layer of isolation.

Then there's social media, where you're bombarded with perfect snapshots of other moms who seem to have it all together. It's a double-edged sword: on one hand, it can help you connect with other moms; on the other, it can make you feel even worse about yourself. Endless feeds of perfectly curated lunches, Montessori toys, and gentle parenting hacks can make you feel like you're failing. Or make you question if you're doing what is truly best for you, and your family… which can be a good thing if it motivates you in a positive way-ha! The guilt piles up until all you want to do is throw your phone in a drawer and forget it exists. And by the way-those moms on social media have an entire team of assistants to make their pages look amazing. They discovered how to ask for help-perhaps we should follow their lead!

Motherhood is hard enough, but when you feel like you're navigating it solo, it's even tougher. And with society's high expectations, and all the ways we're discouraged from asking for help, it's no wonder so many moms are feeling the sting of loneliness. But here's the thing: you're not alone. So many moms are right there with you, feeling exactly the same way. It's just that we don't talk about it nearly enough. Which is why we are talking about it **NOW**!

Why We Need Social Connection

When it comes to feeling good, social connection is right up there with food, water, and sleep. Our interactions with family, friends, colleagues, neighbors—even our digital connections—form the backbone of our emotional and physical well-being. Yet, despite all our tech advances, we're lonelier than ever, and that's especially true for moms.

Humans are wired for connection. Way back in our early

days, being around others wasn't just a nice-to-have; it was crucial for survival. We relied on each other for safety, food, warmth, and community. While we may not need a tribe to fend off wild animals anymore, our brains haven't caught up with the times. We still have this deep-rooted need to connect, even if today we can order everything from groceries to a home gym without stepping foot outside. We may have evolved, but the emotional part of our brain didn't get the memo—and neither did our need for meaningful social connections.

The Physical Toll of Loneliness: Your Heart, Immune System, and More

Loneliness isn't just an emotional drain; it messes with our bodies too. When you're constantly feeling disconnected, it's not just your mind that takes a hit—your heart, immune system, sleep, and even your pain tolerance start to suffer. So how does loneliness impact your physical health?

Cardiovascular Health:
Moms have 27% higher risk of developing heart disease

Immune Function:
Elevated levels of pro-inflammatory cytokines

Sleep Disturbances:
Can't fall asleep or stay asleep

Chronic Pain:
1.8 times more likely to have back pain or fibromyalgia

Cardiovascular Health

Yep, loneliness doesn't just feel like a punch to the heart—it actually puts more strain on it. Research shows that moms who reported persistent loneliness have a whopping **27% higher risk** of developing heart disease. When you're lonely, your body often goes into stress mode, releasing stress hormones that keep your blood pressure elevated. Over time, that constant strain on your heart can lead to serious cardiovascular issues.

Immune Function

When you're lonely, your immune system also starts slacking. Studies have shown that lonely moms have **elevated levels of pro-inflammatory cytokines**, which basically means your body's internal alarm system is always on. Your immune function gets knocked down a few pegs, and suddenly, you're more susceptible to colds, flu, and other infections. It's like your body is too distracted to protect itself properly.

Sleep Disturbances

Loneliness and sleep? A terrible duo. Lonely **moms report** (Malgorzata Witkowska-Zimny et al.) more trouble falling asleep and staying asleep. And when you're not sleeping well, you're setting yourself up for a vicious cycle: lack of sleep worsens loneliness, which messes with sleep even more. It's an exhausting loop that leaves you dragging through the day, which can make you feel even more isolated.

Chronic Pain

As if loneliness wasn't enough of a pain, it can actually cause pain—real, physical pain. Studies have found that moms dealing with loneliness are **1.8 times more likely** (Wilson et al.) to experience chronic pain issues like back pain and fibromyalgia. Loneliness messes with your brain's pain centers, making everything from a sore neck to chronic aches feel more intense.

When loneliness gets its claws into our physical health, it reinforces that cycle of feeling alone, isolated, and unwell. But the good news? Knowing what loneliness does to our bodies is a huge step toward taking back control. There's power in recognizing these impacts, because now, we can start making changes to fight back.

CHAPTER 15

The Power of Mom Communities –The Ultimate Problem Solver

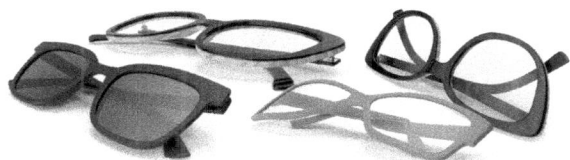

The real devastation? The village that used to help raise kids has practically vanished. We're out here trying to do it all. Without grandparents nearby, without a tight-knit community, and often without even a break to pee alone. Newsflash: we weren't meant to parent in isolation. Raising tiny humans is a team sport, and right now, too many moms are stuck playing solo. It's time to rebuild that village because doing this alone? That was never the plan.

A strong mom community isn't just nice to have, it's a game changer. Having support lightens our stress load, makes parenting easier, and helps us approach our role with more optimism. Studies show that mothers with more support feel happier and more optimistic about parenthood in general.

Here are some ideas on where to find a community that's calling your name:

> ▶ My online community at thereginasteele.com
> ▶ Local gym classes
> ▶ Local mom groups based on interest
> ▶ Volunteer at kids schools
> ▶ Volunteer through kids activities
> ▶ Host potlucks with neighbors or kids school friends

Moms that are surrounded by community often experience:

Lower stress levels – Feeling supported allows moms to connect emotionally with their children without being emotionally drained themselves.

Stronger mental health – Community support acts as a stress buffer, reducing depression, anxiety, and feelings of isolation.

Increased resilience – Surrounding ourselves with an awesome group of other moms **makes navigating challenges more manageable**.

With young moms being more susceptible to high-stress levels, having a community that helps reduce their stress can **positively impact both the mom** and child's well-being. So, instead of asking, "What can I do to help?"—just start doing something! We all see what moms do every day, so step in and make their load lighter.

Longevity Hack: Your Social Circle is a Lifeline

If you thought the secret to a longer, healthier life was just kale smoothies and hitting the gym, think again. Research shows that strong friendships can add years to your life, just as much as quitting smoking or exercising regularly. Let that sink in: your ride-or-die best friend might just be keeping you alive *literally*.

Why? Because humans were never meant to do life alone. The modern obsession with self-sufficiency has left too many moms drowning in stress, pretending we don't need help, while secretly longing for the kind of deep, supportive friendships that make life feel *lighter*.

Friends don't just make life more fun, they protect us from the insidious effects of loneliness, which has been linked to everything from depression to heart disease. Stress-related illnesses? Anxiety? Burnout? A solid social circle acts as a buffer, shielding us from the worst of it.

Motherhood is hard enough without trying to be an island. It's time to rebuild the village.

**Belonging and Self-Worth:
The Power of Just One True Friend**

Here's the truth: you don't need a massive friend group. You just need at least one person you trust completely.

Loneliness isn't just an emotional burden, it's a full-blown health risk. Studies have shown that social isolation is as harmful as smoking 15 cigarettes a day. Let that sink in.

Having even one trusted confidant, someone you can vent

to, laugh with, and ugly-cry in front of, can:

Reduce symptoms of depression and anxiety

Boost self-esteem (because someone actually sees and values you)

Make life's challenges feel more manageable

Motherhood can be isolating, especially when you're surrounded by people but still feel like no one *really* gets what you're going through. But when you have a safe space to be honest, vent, and be seen? It's life-changing.

Friendship isn't just *nice to have*, it's a mental health necessity.

Stress Busters: Friends Are Nature's Best Anxiety Medication

Ever notice how a conversation with a good friend can instantly lift your mood? That's not just in your head (well, technically it is, but *biochemically* speaking).

Social connection literally lowers cortisol levels, the stress hormone that, when chronically high, can wreck your health.

When life gets overwhelming (which, let's be honest, is *every day* for moms), nothing beats a friend who understands:

They help us laugh at the chaos. (Because sometimes, if you don't laugh, you'll cry.)

They provide validation. ("Oh, your toddler also threw their food at the dog? Good. It's not just mine.")

They bring a fresh perspective. ("Maybe, just *maybe*, you're not failing. Maybe you're just tired.")

A 2023 study found that women who have strong friendships report significantly lower levels of stress, anxiety, and depression compared to those who don't. So before you reach for another cup of coffee or a stress snack, try texting your best friend instead.

Friendship: the original therapy session, but free (and usually with snacks).

Brain Boost and Healthier Habits: How Your Tribe Shapes Your Life

Motherhood is not meant to be done alone.

Yet, thanks to modern culture, moms are expected to be self-sufficient, independent, and capable of handling *everything* without help. And the result? A loneliness epidemic.

The reality? We need our people. We need friends who will text us, "I'm bringing you coffee because I know your toddler woke up at 5 AM." We need a support system that says, "You don't have to do this alone." We need relationships that remind us we're *more than just moms.*

So if you feel isolated, it's not you, it's the system that made motherhood a solo sport when it was always meant to be a team effort.

HOW TO ADDRESS LONELINESS IN MOTHERHOOD

Speak Up About Your Feelings

It's easy to withdraw when you're feeling lonely, but keeping it bottled up only makes things worse. Sharing how you're feeling—even if it's awkward—can be a huge relief. Start with your partner. They might not realize how isolated you feel. You could say something like:

> "I'm feeling lonely. It seems like all my relationships have changed, and I'm struggling to know what to do about it. I know you're here, but I still feel disconnected. Can we talk about what I need right now?"

Not ready to talk to your partner? Try confiding in a friend or writing your feelings down. Journaling can help you get clarity on what you're experiencing, which makes it easier to communicate with those who support you.

Embrace Changes in Friendships

Motherhood shifts your social landscape. As you move into this new phase, you might lose some friends and gain others. While it can be hard to let go, finding like-minded moms who are also juggling kids can make a world of difference. Imagine having friends who understand that your plans are subject to change based on nap schedules and snack emergencies. It's liberating!

If you'd like to keep non-parent friends in your life, start by letting them know how you're feeling. They might not realize that maintaining your friendship has become a delicate balancing act. It's okay to say something like:

"I'm feeling lonely and torn. I want to be there for my kids, but I also want to keep our friendship strong. Both are important to me. Can we brainstorm how we can make it work? Your support would mean so much."

Let Go of Unrealistic Expectations

It's tempting to think you have to do everything perfectly, but here's a newsflash: Nobody has it all together. Even if it looks that way online, it's just not true. The research shows that **when moms see more realistic depictions of motherhood,** they feel less lonely. So give yourself permission to break out of the Supermom mold.

Your baby will be fine if they skip a nap because you wanted to catch up with a friend. If you leave a bottle of formula with a sitter for a much-needed date night, guess what? The world will keep spinning. And I know you feel like you're throwing a burden onto others, but grandparents want to help-and it is so so good for them. Your happiness and well-being matter, and they have a huge impact on your kids' happiness and well-being, too. Be kind to yourself; nobody's judging you harder than you are.

Talk to a Professional

Moms are superheroes, but that doesn't mean you can't have some backup. If you've tried everything, or you're just too exhausted to try anything, talking to a professional can give you the boost you need. Feeling lonely isn't a reflection of your worth as a mom; it's a sign that you need some extra TLC. You're not powerless, and you're not broken.

If you're ready for more support, consider reaching out to a therapist or counselor. You can even find specialized resources through **Postpartum Support International** [or any resource you trust]. Or if you're looking for an entire overhaul or a "new lifestyle", I am just a click away. Integrative Health coaching is such an amazing booster for moms that need to inject some vitality into the blah-ness of life. Just remember: you deserve support, too.

Loneliness might feel like it's a part of the mom gig, but it doesn't have to be the forever part. We've tackled the tough truths here because you deserve to know you're not alone in feeling alone. And just by acknowledging it, you're already taking steps to beat it. So, yes, sometimes motherhood can feel like an isolating island, but there's a whole world out there, and a whole community of moms who get it—who get you. We're all in this together, navigating the mess, the magic, and everything in between.

So let's toss the isolation aside and lean into the connection, sisterhood, and support that's waiting for us. After all, moms don't just make the world go 'round; we make it better. And we're here to remind each other of that, every single day.

BREAKING THE CYCLE OF LONELINESS: FINDING YOUR PEOPLE

Loneliness in motherhood is real, but the good news? You don't have to stay stuck in it. Community isn't just a nice-to-have; it's essential for our well-being. So, let's talk about how to break out of isolation and find your people.

Breaking the Cycle of Loneliness:
Finding Your People

Step 1: Acknowledge That You Need Connection

It sounds simple, but the first step is recognizing that loneliness isn't just a personal failing—it's a universal experience in motherhood. Give yourself permission to say, "I need more support."

Step 2: Get Out of Your Comfort Zone

The hardest part? Taking that first step. If making mom friends feels like dating all over again, that's because it kind of is. But connection won't happen unless you put yourself out there. Join a local mom's group, say hi to another mom at the park, or even comment on a social media post. A small effort can spark a big connection.

Step 3: Find the Right Community

Not all mom groups are created equal. Some might feel cliquey, while others are your perfect match. Here are real-life communities where moms are thriving:

► Peanut App – Like Tinder, but for mom friends.

► MOPS (Mothers of Preschoolers) – Faith-based and super supportive.

► Fit4Mom – Workouts + other moms = win-win.

► Local Facebook Groups – A great way to find moms in your area.

► Library Storytime & Kids' Classes – An easy way to meet other moms without forced conversation.

Step 4: Make the First Move

If you meet a mom you click with, don't wait for her to reach out. Suggest a coffee date, a park meetup, or a walk. It feels awkward at first, but most moms are in the same boat—they're just waiting for someone else to make the first move.

Step 5: Cultivate Your Friendships
Friendships take effort. Send the text. Check in. Even if you're busy, small gestures keep connections alive. Remember: your people are out there—you just have to find them.

You're Not Alone

Motherhood can feel isolating, but you don't have to do it alone. The support you need is out there, and connection is closer than you think. You deserve community, laughter, and friendships that make the hard days easier. So go find your people, you're worth it.

What Comes Next?

Moms, you've just taken in a mountain of wisdom. You're armed with insights that can change not only your life but also the lives of those you love most. Let's face it: this world needs strong, empowered moms like you—beacons who can shine a light on a better way forward. You're the ones holding it all together, day in and day out, and whether you realize it or not, your strength and resilience are the foundation our society is built on. Armed with this new knowledge, you're not just surviving; you're thriving, ready to take on the challenges and joys that come your way.

And guess what? You're not doing this alone. There's an army of moms out there—your community, your tribe—cheering you on every step of the way. You've got a massive support network ready to lift you up when you need it, to laugh with you, to cry with you, and to celebrate every hard-won victory. So, let's move forward together, moms. Let's take what we've learned, set our intentions, and create lives for ourselves and our families that radiate health, joy, and resilience. This is your time to rise, and the best is yet to come.

CHAPTER 16

Your Path to a Healthier, Saner Motherhood

So, here we are. You've made it through 15 chapters of call-ing out the nonsense, peeling back the layers of societal B.S., and realizing that, yes, modern motherhood is designed to break us if we don't fight back. But here's the thing: you are fighting back. By simply being here, reading this, absorb-ing these truths, and questioning the status quo, you're already taking the first step toward a healthier, saner version of moth-erhood.

And now? Now it's time to take action.

Let's Get One Thing Straight: You're Not the Problem

If there's one takeaway I need you to tattoo onto your heart, it's this: You are not the problem. The unrealistic expectations? The medical system that dismisses you? The pressure to be everything to everyone? Those are the problems. And trying to "push through" and "handle it" the way society expects is the equivalent of duct-taping your car's check engine light and hoping for the best. Spoiler alert: it doesn't work.

But here's the good news: you don't need to overhaul your entire life in one day.

We're going to take small, sustainable steps toward better health, better balance, and actual joy, not just survival mode. This isn't about making you feel like there's one more thing on your to-do list. It's about empowering you to reclaim control in ways that feel doable and real.

THE MAGIC OF SMALL CHANGES

Ever hear that saying, *small hinges swing big doors*? Turns out, that applies to literally everything in life, including your health, mindset, and happiness.

We're not here for massive, unsustainable shifts that last for two weeks and then crash harder than a toddler skipping a nap. We're here for small, consistent choices that build up over time. Because here's the truth: you don't need a major life overhaul. You just need a shift.

Consider this:

▶ **Five minutes of deep breathing** can lower your stress levels faster than scrolling Instagram in a panic spiral.

▶ **Drinking one extra glass of water** a day can improve your energy levels (because, shocker, dehydration makes you feel like crap).

▶ **Swapping one ultra-processed snack** for a whole food

option can help stabilize your mood and blood sugar.

► **Getting outside for ten minutes** a day can help regulate your circadian rhythm and improve your sleep.

Tiny changes lead to big results.

YOU'VE GOT THIS

This book isn't here to tell you "just try harder." This book is here to tell you that you're already trying harder than you should have to. The system wasn't built to support moms, but that doesn't mean we can't reclaim our health, sanity, and joy, on our own terms.

So here's my challenge to you: pick ONE of these protocols and start today. Just one. Not everything at once. Not a full lifestyle transformation overnight. Just one small step in the direction of the life you deserve.

Because you deserve to feel good. You deserve to be supported. And you deserve to be more than just someone who survives motherhood, you deserve to thrive in it.

Now, let's get started. The Protocols are where we make this real.

Are you ready? Let's go.

PART 02

Self Healing Protocols

The Mom Health Pillars:
Holding You Up When Coffee Fails

Welcome to the part of the book where you become the head practitioner of your own health. Yes, you read that right. YOU. Before you panic and assume I'm telling you to ghost your doctor and rely on Google University, take a breath. I'm not here to tell you to toss out all professional medical advice. But I *am* here to hand you back the reins of your own well-being because, let's be honest, too many of us have been conditioned to ignore our own gut instincts when it comes to our health.

After diving into everything in the first part of this book, you now have a clearer picture of why modern motherhood has us all feeling like overworked, under-rested lab rats in a never-ending experiment. I hit that wall too. I got tired of prescriptions being the first (and sometimes only) solution handed to me. I got sick of being told, *"That's just part of being a mom,"* like exhaustion, depletion, and chronic stress were normal. So, I took matters into my own hands.

I read. I researched. I experimented. I worked with professionals who actually saw me as a whole person rather than a walking set of symptoms. And, most importantly, I worked with other moms who were struggling just like me. Through my own experience, as a mom, an integrative health coach, and someone who got fed up with feeling like crap, I built this health plan. Not based on trends, not based on what the wellness industry says you *should* do, but based on what actually worked for me and the countless moms I've worked with.

This isn't a one-size-fits-all approach. It's a blueprint that allows you to build your foundation, one pillar at a time. These pillars of motherhood health—nutrition, movement, sleep, stress management, and mental well-being—are the things that made the biggest impact in real life. Not in some perfect, Instagram-filtered version of motherhood, but in the chaotic, messy, *real* version we live every day. And trust me, when you start implementing even a few of these practices, you'll see a ripple effect, not just in yourself, but in your family, your home, and beyond. When your energy shifts, so does everything around you.

HERE'S HOW THIS SECTION WORKS

This section is designed to take the guesswork out of creating a healthier, more balanced life. I know you're busy, I know your brain is already running on overdrive, and I know the last thing you need is another *complicated* health plan that makes you feel like a failure before you even start. That's why these protocols are simple, actionable, and mom-approved.

Here's how each protocol is laid out so you can actually use it, without having to decode medical jargon or waste time figuring out where to start.

1. Why This Protocol Matters

Before diving into the *how*, we'll start with the *why*. Because let's be honest, if you don't know why something is important, it's way easier to shove it to the bottom of your priority list (and jam it underneath all the random keys in your kitchen junk drawer). This section will break down exactly why this protocol is a game-changer for your health and how it fits into the bigger picture of feeling like *you* again.

2. What To Expect: The Possibilities

Let's talk results. This section will cover what's possible when you start integrating this protocol. Better sleep? More energy? Less mom rage? A sudden ability to function before coffee? This is your sneak peek at the benefits so you can actually look forward to what's ahead.

3. Tools & Materials That May Come in Handy

Here's your go-to for anything that might make this process easier. From kitchen essentials for nutrition protocols to sleep gadgets for better rest, this section covers anything that can help you win at this whole *taking-care-of-yourself* thing. (And no, none of them require spending a fortune or reorganizing your entire life.)

4. The Checklist—Because What Mom Doesn't Love a Checklist?

This is your quick, no-fluff rundown of what needs to happen. Think of it as your health to-do list, minus the overwhelm. Whether you're a "write it down so I can cross it off" kind of mom or you just need a straightforward guide, this section is here to make your life a little easier.

5. Actionable Steps—A.K.A. The Actual Protocol

This is where the magic happens. No vague advice, no confusing wellness buzzwords. Just clear, step-by-step instructions that tell you *exactly* what to do. Each protocol is broken down into easy, doable steps that you can actually fit into your already packed schedule.

6. Example 7 Day Plan—Just for Ideas

I know that every mom's day looks different, so this is not about rigid routines or unattainable schedules. Instead, this section gives you a flexible blueprint so you can see how this protocol might fit into real life (yes, even *your* real life).

7. FAQs—I Know You Have Questions, So Here Are My Answers

This section tackles common concerns, roadblocks, and "what if" scenarios that might pop up as you go. Whether it's "What if I miss a day?" or "How do I get my family on board?"—I've got you covered.

YOU WILL FIND THE FOLLOWING TREASURES IN THE APPENDIX IN THE BACK OF THE BOOK:

Real Talk Resources —Your Go-To for Extra Support

Need more evidence before jumping in? I totally get it—I've spent this whole book telling you to *question everything*. So, in the spirit of doing your own research, here are some trusted websites, studies, and resources to help you dig deeper. Whether you're looking for extra guidance, scientific backup, or just a little reassurance when motivation wavers, this section has you covered.

Additional Material—"Helpers"

These are the extra goodies. Cheat sheets, journal prompts, tracking sheets, or simple hacks that make these protocols even easier to implement. Think of this section as your bonus round, where you get extra support to stay on track.

This is your toolkit. You get to use it however it best serves you. And the best part? You don't have to do it all at once. Even small changes can yield massive results.

So, let's get started. Your health (and your sanity) are about to get the upgrade they deserve. And in case you need a recap from the first part of the book, or you're just too busy being mom, here's the **TL;DR** (too long; didn't read) version:

MOM'S QUICK START GUIDE TO SANITY

1. NUTRITION: EAT LIKE YOU ACTUALLY MATTER

  ▶ Crowd out the junk—don't obsess over removing foods, just add more whole foods in.

  ▶ Balance your blood sugar to stop feeling like an unstable mess (protein + fiber at every meal!).

  ▶ Hydrate! Dehydration = exhaustion.

  ▶ Food affects mood. Eat like someone who deserves to feel good.

165

2. MOVEMENT: YOU DON'T HAVE TO "WORK OUT" TO MOVE YOUR BODY

► Walk more—even 10 minutes a day makes a difference.

► Stretch, dance, clean with extra energy. It all counts.

► Find something fun. If you hate it, you won't do it. Period.

3. SLEEP: PRIORITIZE REST LIKE YOUR SANITY DEPENDS ON IT (BECAUSE IT DOES)

► Nighttime routine matters. Dim the lights, cut the screens.

► Your bed is for sleep (not revenge-scrolling TikTok at 1 AM).

► Improve sleep quality, not just quantity. Magnesium, blackout curtains, and a consistent bedtime make a huge difference.

4. MENTAL HEALTH: GET OFF THE MARTYR TRAIN

► Ask for help. Not a weakness—a power move.

► Boundaries are a full sentence. "No" is not a dirty word.

► Therapy is self-care. If you need it, get it.

5. COMMUNITY: FIND YOUR PEOPLE

► Motherhood isn't meant to be done alone. Join a group, reconnect with a friend, or talk to another mom at the park.

► Ditch toxic relationships. If they drain you, they gotta go.

► Be intentional about connection. Even a 5-minute voice note to a friend can lift you up.

Purpose: Rediscovering YOU

Why This Protocol Matters

Purpose isn't just some fluffy, motivational-poster concept. It's as essential as sleep, food, and that first glorious sip of coffee in the morning. According to Alan Rozanski, Professor of Medicine at Mount Sinai, purpose is a fundamental psychological need, just like eating and sleeping. Research even suggests that people with a strong sense of purpose live longer, are healthier, and experience less stress (so basically, purpose is the secret weapon of sanity).

But here's the catch. Mom-life has a way of swallowing up everything else. It's easy to get lost in the daily grind of snack-making, crisis-managing, and laundry-folding (or at least laundry-moving-from-one-pile-to-another). This protocol is about reclaiming what makes you, YOU. It's not about adding more to your to-do list, it's about creating space for what truly fulfills you.

So, squash the guilt. Prioritizing your purpose isn't selfish, it's necessary. When you're engaged in something meaningful, you're a happier, healthier mom, partner, and human. That's not just good for you, it's good for everyone around you.

WHAT TO EXPECT: THE POSSIBILITIES

When you reconnect with purpose, amazing things happen:

Less Stress: Purpose helps you focus on what actually matters, lowering stress hormones (goodbye, cortisol overload).

Better Mental Clarity: When you're aligned with what excites you, brain fog lifts, and decision-making gets easier.

Stronger Emotional Resilience: Life's setbacks won't knock you down as easily when you're rooted in something meaningful.

Healthier Habits: Purpose-driven people make better choices: exercise, nutrition, and sleep improve **without forcing it**.

More Energy & Motivation: When you're doing what lights you up, you actually want to get out of bed (most days).

Stronger Immune System: Studies show a link between purpose and fewer sick days. Science says, **"Find your why, avoid the flu."**

Lower Risk of Anxiety & Depression: Feeling connected to a purpose reduces the mental health rollercoaster.

Improved Heart Health: A clear sense of purpose = lower blood pressure and a healthier heart.

Better Relationships: Purpose-driven people cultivate stronger social connections.

Enhanced Self-Worth: Because you're so much more than "just Mom."

If any of these sound too good to be true, that's exactly why this matters. The ripple effect of rediscovering your purpose is real.

TOOLS & MATERIALS THAT MAY COME IN HANDY

You don't need much, but these can help make the process smoother:

Journals & Reflection Tools

The Five-Minute Journal: Quick daily gratitude and purpose prompts

The Artist's Way Morning Pages Journal: A creative approach to rediscovering what excites you

Promptly Journals: Tailored for life transitions, including motherhood.

Planners & Digital Organizers

Passion Planner: A goal-oriented planner with room for weekly reflections.

Cozi Family Organizer App: Keep track of family AND personal goals.

Trello: Organize purpose-driven tasks in an easy-to-use format.

Podcasts & Books for Inspiration

The Purpose Show (Allie Casazza): A deep dive into decluttering life for meaning.

Big Magic (Elizabeth Gilbert): Embracing creativity and purpose without fear.

Start With Why (Simon Sinek): Helps define personal "why"

Community & Accountability

Peanut App A social networking app for moms looking to connect.

Meetup.com Find purpose-driven groups or workshops

The Mom Reset Yep, my online community is here to help you stay motivated and connected!

Having one or two of these tools in your arsenal makes this whole process easier. Is it required, no! So, if you are already burning on fumes, just grab whatever random stuff you have laying around. It all works the same.

THE CHECKLIST

❏ **Journal & Reflect**
Write down thoughts, dreams, and insights

❏ **Schedule one weekly "me-time" session**
Even if it's just 15 minutes

❏ **Try a new hobby or interest**
Explore without pressure

❏ **Set one small, achievable goal**
Something that excites you

❏ **Connect with a purpose buddy**
Because accountability makes it stick

Small, consistent actions make a big impact over time. Pick one of the above, and go from there. Need to wait a week in between each addition…totally fine, but stretch any farther than that, you may need to work one on one with me-ha! I'll get ya moving!

ACTIONABLE STEPS

QUICK GUIDE

Step 1   Reflect on What Matters

Step 2   Set a Mini-Goal

Step 3   Build a Purposeful Routine

Step 4   Find a Purpose Buddy

Step 5   Experiment & Explore

Step 6   Reflect & Adjust

STEP 1: REFLECT ON WHAT MATTERS TO YOU

Take 10-15 minutes to journal about:

When do I feel happiest?

What activities make me lose track of time?

What did I love doing as a kid?

If I had an extra hour every day, what would I do?

No judgment, no overthinking, just let the answers flow.

Action: Pick ONE thing that excites you and write it down.

STEP 2: SET A MINI-GOAL

Based on your reflections, set one small goal (ex: 10 minutes of journaling a day, signing up for a class, or reconnecting with an old hobby).

Keep it realistic and manageable, this isn't about adding stress!

Action: Write your goal down and set a specific day to start.

STEP 3: BUILD A PURPOSEFUL ROUTINE

Schedule at least one "me-time" session each week.

Use this time for anything that fuels you: reading, writing, painting, exercising, whatever makes you feel alive.

Protect this time like you protect nap time.

Action: Add this "me-time" to your calendar and stick to it.

STEP 4: FIND A PURPOSE BUDDY

Reach out to a friend, fellow mom, or join a community

Schedule bi-weekly check-ins for support and motivation.

 Action: Send a message to someone today and set up your first check-in.

STEP 5: EXPERIMENT & EXPLORE

Try something new: sign up for a class, start a project, volunteer, or just dabble in a hobby.

No pressure to "get it right", this is about fun and self-discovery.

Action: Block off 15-20 minutes this week to try something new.

STEP 6: REFLECT & ADJUST

At the end of each week, ask:
What did I enjoy the most?
What felt meh?
What do I want to try next?

Adjust your goals and routines accordingly.

Action: Celebrate small wins. Progress is progress.

By following these steps, you'll be gradually building a routine around your sense of purpose, one that's sustainable, enjoyable, and uniquely yours. This protocol isn't about adding more to your plate but about finding those moments that make you feel more like you.

EXAMPLE 7-DAY PLAN

(Because Purpose Doesn't Just Appear. You Create It!)

This schedule is designed to be realistic for busy moms. Each day includes a small, intentional step that fits into everyday life. No massive time commitments, just bite-sized actions that add up over time.

Day 1	REFLECT & SET A MINI-GOAL (10-15 MIN)
Objective:	Start the week by reconnecting with yourself and setting a small, achievable goal.
Activity:	Take 10-15 minutes (nap time, early morning, bedtime, whenever works).
	Reflect on these prompts (choose one or two):
	► What makes me feel the most alive?
	► What did I love doing as a child?
	► If I could spend a day doing anything, what would it be?
	Set one small goal for the week (e.g., "I'll spend 10 minutes journaling each day" or "I'll explore a new hobby").
	Mindset Tip: Purpose isn't about finding yourself, it's about creating yourself.

Day 2	PURPOSEFUL "ME-TIME" (10-15 MIN)
Objective:	Do one small activity that brings you joy, without overthinking it.

Activity: Choose an activity that lights you up:

▶ Journal

▶ Read a chapter of a book

▶ Sketch or doodle

▶ Play music

▶ Sit outside in silence

▶ Do a creative hobby (knitting, writing, crafting)

Set a timer for 10-15 minutes and let yourself enjoy it.

Mindset Tip: Purpose doesn't need to be "productive." If it makes you feel good, it's valid.

Day 3	CHECK-IN WITH A PURPOSE BUDDY (15-20 MIN)

Objective: Do one small activity that brings you joy, without overthinking it.

Activity: Choose an activity that lights you up:

▶ Call, text, or meet up with a friend who gets it.

▶ Share what you're exploring and ask them what excite them.

If you don't have a "purpose buddy" yet, join a supportive online group.

Mindset Tip: Having accountability makes purpose stick. Find someone to cheer you on.

Day 4	EXPLORE SOMETHING NEW (15-20 MIN)

Objective: Step slightly out of your routine and try something new, no pressure.

Activity: Pick something you've **always been curious about**:

▶ Try a new recipe

▶ Watch a TED Talk on something inspiring

▶ Write a short poem or journal entry

▶ Sign up for a free online class or webinar

▶ Browse hobbies and interests on Pinterest

No perfection required, just explore.

Mindset Tip: Purpose isn't about having all the answers, it's about staying curious.

Day 5	REFLECT & ADJUST (15-20 MIN)

Objective: Look back at the week and see what clicked (and what didn't).

Activity: Write down:

► What did I enjoy most this week?

► What felt "meh"?

► What would I like to explore more?

Adjust next week's focus based on what felt good.

Mindset Tip: It's okay to change direction. Purpose is a moving target.

Day 6	DO SOMETHING THAT FILLS YOUR CUP (20-30 MIN)

Objective: Carve out intentional time for something that feels like YOU.

Activity: Choose one of the following:

► Go for a walk (alone or with a podcast)

► Take yourself out for coffee

► Work on a fun project (writing, painting, DIY)

► Meditate or practice deep breathing

► Listen to an inspiring podcast

Plan something exciting for the future (a class, trip, or personal goal)

Mindset Tip: If you never take time for you, who will?

177

Day 7	CELEBRATE & SET NEXT STEPS (15-20 MIN)
Objective:	End the week by celebrating small wins and setting new intentions.
Activity:	Write down three wins from the week (even tiny ones!). Answer these prompts:
	► What did I learn about myself this week?
	► What's one thing I want to continue exploring?
	► What small step can I take next week?
	If you're feeling extra fancy, make a **vision board** (digital or paper) of things that **excite you**.
	Mindset Tip: Growth isn't about giant leaps, it's about small, consistent steps. Focus on the experience.

This 7-day schedule is meant to be flexible—if you miss a day, no big deal. The key is momentum.

Start small. Stay curious. Enjoy the process

By the end of the week, you'll have: More clarity about what excites you, A sense of accomplishment (even if it's tiny), A foundation for rediscovering purpose.

You got this.

FAQS

Q: Isn't it selfish to focus on my purpose with all my mom responsibilities?

A: Nope! Actually, science says it's as essential as getting enough sleep (which, let's face it, is already rare enough). When you nurture yourself, everyone wins—you'll have more patience, energy, and even creativity to handle whatever motherhood throws your way (yes, even glitter).

Q: What if I don't know what my purpose is?

A: That's totally okay. Purpose doesn't always come with flash-

178

ing neon lights. Think of it as an ongoing experiment—try new things, revisit old passions, and give yourself permission to be curious. Purpose is like a great pair of jeans; you'll know it fits when you find it.

Q: I can barely make time to shower—how am I supposed to find time for purpose?

A: We get it! This isn't about adding hours of "me-time" to your schedule; it's about adding small, intentional moments. Start with just 5-10 minutes a day doing something meaningful to you. Purpose doesn't require a major time commitment; it's the little sparks of joy and fulfillment that make a difference.

Q: What if I start a new hobby or project and then totally lose interest?

A: No big deal! Purpose is allowed to evolve. Just like toddlers go from loving peas to refusing them in a week, you're allowed to change what interests you. Each experience adds a new layer to your life, so embrace the adventure and don't worry about "sticking with it" unless it truly brings you joy.

Q: How do I explain to my kids why I need time for myself?

A: Try something like, "Mom needs time to recharge her superpowers so she can be the best mom for you!" Kids are amazing at understanding that grown-ups need a break, too. Plus, you're setting an example that self-care is important.

Q: I feel guilty doing things just for myself. Any tips for ditching the mom guilt?

A: Ah, the classic mom guilt! Here's a thought: When you take care of yourself, you're teaching your kids that moms are people too. So next time guilt creeps in, remind yourself you're showing them the importance of self-love and balance. Plus, who doesn't want a mom who's happier and less stressed? (Especially if you have infants, toddlers, or teens-haha)

Q: Does purpose always have to be something "productive"?

A: Absolutely not! Purpose isn't about productivity; it's about fulfillment. If lying in the grass watching clouds fills you up, then that's purposeful. If your soul feels happier after an hour of doodling or listening to music, that's valuable too. Purpose is about what makes you feel alive, not what looks productive.

Q: I tried journaling, and all I wrote was "I'm tired" ten times. Am I doing this wrong?

A: Nope, that's a totally valid entry! In fact, it's probably the most honest journal prompt out there. Sometimes, simply acknowledging your exhaustion is the first step to figuring out what you need. Don't worry about "perfect" reflections—just keep showing up and let your thoughts flow. The insights will come. (And go lay down to recharge for 10-15 minutes!)

Q: How do I handle days when I just don't feel like doing any of this?

A: Be kind to yourself. Some days, the most purposeful thing you can do is give yourself a break. Purpose doesn't mean being on a mission every single day—it's okay to have off days, lazy days, or "just survive" days. Rest and recharge, then jump back in when you're ready.

Q: Can my purpose change over time?

A: Absolutely! Purpose is a moving target. (Is there an echo in here?) Who you are and what lights you up can shift as you grow, experience new things, and move through different stages of motherhood. Purpose isn't a one-and-done—it evolves with you. Embrace the journey and let your purpose change as you do!

Think of purpose as your body's personal bodyguard. It helps keep those stress hormones in check (you know, the ones that spike when your kid announces their science project is due tomorrow), boosts your immune system (essential for surviving preschool germs), and even helps your heart stay stronger. Plus - and this is my favorite part - **purposeful mommas tend to make better lifestyle choices**. They're more likely to actually use that gym membership instead of just keeping the card as a fancy bookmark, eat more veggies, and maybe not finish that entire bottle of wine on Wednesday night.

Nutrition: Fueling Your Body Without the Overwhelm

Nutrition & Nourishment: Eating for Energy and Sanity

Why This Protocol Matters

Moms are nutrient-deprived superheroes, surviving on coffee, leftover crusts, and whatever snack their toddler rejected. If you've ever thought, "Why am I so exhausted all the time?"—this is why. Poor nutrition leads to blood sugar crashes, mood swings, and a constant energy deficit. The goal isn't perfection; it's about eating real, nutrient-dense foods that fit into your life without the stress of extreme diets or food guilt. If you want to feel good, have more energy, and stop riding the sugar-crash roller coaster, this is where you start.

What To Expect: The Possibilities

Here's what happens when you shift to real, whole foods:

More Energy: No more surviving on caffeine fumes

Better Mental Clarity: Say goodbye to the "What did I come in here for?" moments

Balanced Blood Sugar: Less moodiness, fewer cravings

Stronger Immune System: Fewer sick days (for you AND the kids)

Better Digestion: Less bloating, more ahem regularity

Healthier Weight Balance: Your metabolism actually works

Radiant Skin & Hair: Because glowing is always better than exhausted

The best part? You don't have to overhaul your entire kitchen overnight. Small changes add up fast.

TOOLS & MATERIALS THAT MAY COME IN HANDY

You don't need a full kitchen makeover, but these essentials will make life easier:

Kitchen Basics for Healthy Eating

Non-Toxic Cookware: Ditch Teflon, opt for ceramic, cast iron, or stainless steel

Glass Storage Containers: Because plastic + heat = hormone-disrupting chemicals

High-Powered Blender: For smoothies, soups, and sauces (Vitamix or Ninja)

Air-Tight Food Storage: Keeps bulk pantry staples fresh

Water Filtration System: Tap water is sketchy; upgrade to Berkey or AquaTru

Stock Your Pantry With These Staples

Whole Grains: Quinoa, brown rice, oats

Healthy Fats: Avocado oil, olive oil, coconut oil, ghee

Proteins: Grass-fed meats, wild-caught fish, pasture-raised eggs

Nuts & Seeds: Almonds, walnuts, flax, chia

Legumes: Lentils, chickpeas, black beans

Organic Spices & Herbs: Turmeric, cinnamon, garlic

A well-stocked kitchen makes healthy eating easier. You can find a detailed List in the Appendix in the back of the book.

THE CHECKLIST

- ☐ **Declutter the pantry**
  (Bye-bye, ultra-processed junk)
- ☐ **Stock up on whole, real foods**
- ☐ **Prep easy grab-and-go snacks**
- ☐ **Plan simple meals**
  (no fancy gourmet skills required)
- ☐ **Prep easy grab-and-go snacks**
- ☐ **Prioritize hydration**
  (because coffee isn't water)

Simple. Achievable. Mom-friendly.

Actionable Steps

Are you ready? The following steps will help you build a healthy kitchen step-by-step, making it easy to create balanced meals and maintain healthy eating habits. By following each step, you'll simplify meal prep, reduce stress, and set yourself up for success with nourishing choices that work for you and your family.

NUTRITION QUICK GUIDE

Step 1	Clean & Simplify Your Pantry
Step 2	Stock Up on Whole Foods
Step 3	Fill the Fridge with Fresh, Quality Foods
Step 4	Plan Simple Meals
Step 5	Hydration is Key
Step 6	Snack Smarter
Step 7	Create a Weekly Grocery List & Stick to It

Step 1: Clean & Simplify Your Pantry

Toss the ultra-processed junk. Replace as you go. Stick to ingredients you recognize, fewer than 5 is ideal. Rotate spices & oils. Ditch canola, use avocado, olive, or coconut oil. Use EWG's Dirty Dozen & Clean 15 lists to prioritize organic.

Action: Gradually replace processed foods with real, whole ingredients.

Step 2: Stock Up on Whole Foods

Whole Grains: Quinoa, brown rice, oats, buckwheat.
Legumes: Lentils, chickpeas, black beans.
Nuts & Seeds: Almonds, walnuts, chia, flax.

186

Healthy Fats: Avocado oil, olive oil, coconut oil, ghee.
Protein: Grass-fed meats, pasture-raised eggs, wild-caught fish.

Action: Build a pantry that supports quick, nutrient-dense meals.

Step 3: Fill the Fridge with Fresh, Quality Foods

Vegetables: Load up on leafy greens, root veggies, cruciferous vegetables.
Fruits: Berries, citrus, apples, pears.
Dairy (if tolerated): Grass-fed butter, Greek yogurt, raw cheese.
Proteins: Pasture-raised eggs, organic chicken, grass-fed beef, wild-caught fish.

Action: Wash, chop, and store fresh produce for easy grab-and-go meals.

Step 4: Plan Simple Meals

Batch cook basics: Roast veggies, cook a protein, prep a grain.
Use a recipe rotation: Keep 5-6 go-to meals in rotation
Mix up flavors with sauces: Try tahini, pesto, or Greek yogurt-based dressings.
Make leftovers work: Roasted veggies turns into frittata, grilled chicken turns into salads.

Action: Keep meal prep simple & repeatable, less stress, more ease. Try one of the batch prepping ideas and see how it goes! If one works out, maybe try another, and build on one after another, until you get the hang of prepping. I promise, this will change your life!

Step 5: Hydration is Key

Drink half your body weight in ounces of water daily.
Upgrade hydration: Add lemon, cucumber, or sea salt for electrolytes. Limit caffeine to mornings. Try matcha or herbal tea later in the day.

Action: Keep a water bottle nearby and aim for consistent hydration.

Step 6: Snack Smarter

Pair protein & fiber: Apple + almond butter, Greek yogurt + berries.
Replace chips with crunch: Air-popped popcorn, roasted chickpeas.
DIY energy bites: Oats, nut butter, honey—done.
Choose low-sugar: Bars with <5g sugar, unsweetened nut butters.

Action: Prep easy-to-grab snacks to prevent energy crashes.

Step 7: Create a Weekly Grocery List & Stick to It

Keep a running list: Write down items as they run out
Shop in zones: Stick to the store's perimeter.
Avoid impulse buys: Shop full, not hungry.

Action: Plan meals and shop intentionally to avoid stress. And no, fancy digital checklists and apps are not necessary. A simple piece of paper works quite well.

EXAMPLE 7 DAY PLAN

Day 1	
Breakfast	Greek (or coconut) yogurt bowl with mixed berries, a sprinkle of chia seeds, and a drizzle of honey.

Lunch	Quinoa salad with mixed greens, cherry tomatoes, cucumber, shredded carrots, chickpeas, and a lemon-tahini dressing.
Diner	Sheet-pan roasted chicken thighs with sweet potatoes, bell peppers, and broccoli.
Snacks	Apple slices with almond butter, a handful of mixed nuts.
Hydration	Water infused with lemon slices throughout the day, plus a cup of peppermint tea in the evening.

Day 2

Breakfast	Overnight oats made with almond milk, topped with sliced banana, walnuts, and a sprinkle of cinnamon.
Lunch	Chopped chicken and avocado wrap using a whole-grain tortilla, with lettuce, tomato, and a side of mixed berries.
Diner	Stir-fried tofu or chicken with brown rice and a medley of bell peppers, snap peas, carrots, and broccoli, seasoned with a dash of tamari sauce and sesame seeds
Snacks	Greek yogurt with a handful of blueberries, a few slices of cucumber and bell pepper with hummus.
Hydration	Water infused with cucumber and mint, and a glass of iced hibiscus tea mid-afternoon.

Day 3

Breakfast	Smoothie with spinach, banana, frozen berries, a scoop of almond butter, and a spoonful of flax seeds.
Lunch	Grain bowl with quinoa, roasted chickpeas, mixed greens, shredded carrots, and a tahini dressing.
Diner	Baked salmon with a side of roasted Brussels sprouts and garlic mashed cauliflower.
Snacks	A handful of walnuts, baby carrots with guacamole.
Hydration	Water with lime slices, plus a glass of chamomile tea before bed.

Day 4

Breakfast	Scrambled eggs with spinach and cherry tomatoes, served with a slice of sourdough toast and avocado.
Lunch	Mason jar salad with mixed greens, diced bell peppers, cucumbers, shredded chicken, and a balsamic vinaigrette.
Diner	Lentil and vegetable stew with carrots, celery, potatoes, and spinach, served with a side of sourdough bread.
Snacks	Sliced pear with a few almonds, a small bowl of Greek yogurt with a sprinkle of chia seeds.
Hydration	Water infused with orange slices, and a cup of ginger tea in the evening.

Day 5

Breakfast	Chia pudding made with coconut milk, topped with fresh strawberries and a sprinkle of granola.
Lunch	Leftover lentil and vegetable stew, with a side salad of mixed greens and a light vinaigrette.
Diner	Grilled steak or Cauliflower steak with a side of roasted butternut squash and green beans.
Snacks	Celery sticks with almond butter, a few dried apricots.
Hydration	Water with cucumber slices, plus a glass of lemon balm tea in the afternoon.

Day 6

Breakfast	Oatmeal topped with diced apple, a sprinkle of cinnamon, and chopped pecans.
Lunch	Tuna salad with wild-caught tuna, mixed greens, cherry tomatoes, cucumber, and a drizzle of olive oil and vinegar.
Diner	Zucchini or Spaghetti noodles with marinara sauce, ground turkey, and a sprinkle of parmesan cheese, with a side of steamed broccoli.

| Snacks | A handful of raw cashews, red bell pepper slices with hummus. |
| Hydration | Water infused with fresh basil and lemon, plus a cup of green tea after lunch. |

Day 7	
Breakfast	Smoothie bowl with blended frozen berries, spinach, and a scoop of protein powder, topped with chia seeds and sliced banana.
Lunch	Sweet potato and black bean bowl with quinoa, mixed greens, diced avocado, and salsa.
Diner	Baked cod with roasted carrots, asparagus, and a side of garlic mashed sweet potatoes.
Snacks	Sliced cucumber with hummus, a small bowl of mixed fruit.
Hydration	Water with a few fresh berries for a hint of flavor, and a cup of rooibos tea before bed.

Weekly Summary for Snacks and Hydration:

Aim for a balance of protein, fiber, and healthy fats with each snack. Mix and match fruits (like apple, pear, or berries), veggies (carrots, bell peppers, cucumber), nuts (almonds, walnuts, or cashews), and dips (hummus, almond butter) to keep snacks interesting.

Pre-portion snacks in reusable containers so they're easy to grab when hunger hits.

Hydration Goals:

Drink a full glass of water upon waking and keep a water bottle nearby throughout the day.

Aim to drink water between meals and add variety with

herbal teas or infused water (e.g., lemon, mint, or cucumber).

Include hydrating foods like cucumber, citrus fruits, and watermelon for additional hydration support.

This meal plan emphasizes nutrient-dense, whole foods, making it easy to keep you and your family nourished, satisfied, and hydrated all week long. Adjust portion sizes and specific ingredients based on personal preferences or dietary needs, and feel free to swap meals between days as needed for variety.

BONUS PROTOCOLS & GUIDES FOR SPECIFIC PHASES OF MOTHERHOOD

NUTRITION PROTOCOL FOR MOMS IN THE FERTILITY PHASE

This protocol is designed for moms thinking about conceiving, focusing on a fertility-friendly diet to nourish the body, support hormone balance, and boost overall reproductive health.

Step 1	Prioritize Folate-Rich Foods and Key Nutrients
Step 2	Focus on Organic and Pasture-Raised Foods
Step 3	Limit Alcohol, Caffeine, and Nicotine
Step 4	Add Fertility-Boosting Supplements
Step 5	Include Your Partner in the Nutritional Plan

Step 1: Prioritize Folate-Rich Foods and Key Nutrients

Action: Increase intake of folate-rich foods to support

healthy cell growth and prevent birth defects. Aim for foods like leafy greens, beans, avocados, and citrus fruits. Consider a quality prenatal supplement that includes folic acid, zinc, selenium, omega-3s, vitamin E, and vitamin C to support fertility.

Tips & Hacks:

Choose Folate over Synthetic Folic Acid: Look for natural sources of folate (from foods) or methylfolate in supplements, as they are more easily absorbed by the body.

Go for Bright Colors: Include a variety of colorful fruits and veggies for a full spectrum of antioxidants and vitamins.

Consider Split Dosing: If a prenatal vitamin feels heavy on your stomach, try taking half in the morning and half in the evening.

Healthy Brands to Consider:

Garden of Life: Known for whole-food-based, organic prenatals with methylfolate.

Thorne Research: Offers high-quality prenatal vitamins with essential fertility nutrients.

Nordic Naturals: Provides high-quality omega-3 supplements with DHA, critical for fetal brain development and fertility health.

Step 2: Focus on Organic and Pasture-Raised Foods

Action: Choose organic fruits and vegetables, as well as grass-fed or pasture-raised meat and eggs. This helps limit exposure to pesticides, hormones, and antibiotics that may interfere with hormone balance.

Tips & Hacks:

Prioritize the Dirty Dozen: Use the Environmental Working Group's (EWG) Dirty Dozen list to know which produce to buy organic.

Look for Grass-Fed Labels: Choose grass-fed beef and dairy or pasture-raised eggs for a cleaner source of protein and fats.

Bulk Up with Freezer: Buy organic or pasture-raised meats in bulk and freeze portions for future use, saving both time and money.

Healthy Brands to Consider:

Vital Farms: Known for pasture-raised eggs that are hormone and antibiotic-free.

ButcherBox: Delivers grass-fed, pasture-raised meats directly to your door.

Thrive Market: Offers a variety of organic produce, pantry staples, and meats for a fertility-focused diet.

Step 3: Limit Alcohol, Caffeine, and Nicotine

Action: Avoid alcohol, caffeine, and nicotine as much as possible, as all three can decrease fertility and negatively impact hormone balance.

Tips & Hacks:

Switch to Decaf or Herbal Teas: If you're a coffee lover, gradually switch to decaf or try herbal teas that support hormone health, such as raspberry leaf or peppermint.

Explore Mocktails: For social events, try non-alcoholic alternatives like sparkling water with a splash of juice and a slice of lime.

Create New Habits: Replace caffeine and alcohol with fertility-friendly drinks like green smoothies, which are rich in folate and antioxidants.

Healthy Brands to Consider:

Reishi Tea: Organic, caffeine-free herbal teas that support hydration and relaxation.

Four Sigmatic: Known for caffeine-free, adaptogenic drinks, which can support stress management.

LaCroix or Spindrift: Sparkling waters with no added sugars for a refreshing, caffeine-free beverage.

Step 4: Add Fertility-Boosting Supplements

Action: In addition to folate, consider adding supplements like zinc, selenium, omega-3s, vitamin E, and vitamin C to boost fertility. These nutrients help improve egg quality, balance hormones, and reduce inflammation.

Tips & Hacks:

Consider a Multivitamin with Prenatal Support: A good prenatal multivitamin often covers these essentials, making it easy to get your nutrients in one place.

Divide Doses with Your Partner: If your partner is also taking supplements, you can align your schedules to make taking them a habit together.

Omega-3 Sources: If you prefer food sources, add fatty fish like salmon twice a week or incorporate flax seeds and chia seeds into your diet.

Healthy Brands to Consider:

Garden of Life MyKind Organics: Offers a whole-food-based prenatal with folate, zinc, and vitamin C.

Nordic Naturals: Provides high-quality omega-3 supplements with both DHA and EPA for fertility support.

Pure Encapsulations: A reputable brand for zinc and selenium supplements.

Step 5: Include Your Partner in the Nutritional Plan

Action: Remember, about 40% of fertility challenges can be on the partner's side. Encourage your partner to also focus on a nutrient-rich diet and consider supplements like zinc, vitamin C, calcium, and vitamin D.

Tips & Hacks:

Create Shared Healthy Meals: Make meals that are nutrient-dense for both of you, like leafy green salads with salmon, nuts, and a squeeze of lemon for added vitamin C.

Shared Supplement Routine: Take supplements together to help create a routine and make it easy to remember.

Focus on Whole Foods: Incorporate fertility-boosting foods into your shared meals, like nuts, seeds, lean meats, and dark leafy greens.

Healthy Brands to Consider *(cause we aren't the only ones responsible for making a baby)*:

Rainbow Light Men's One Multivitamin: A comprehensive multivitamin that covers essential nutrients for male fertility.

MegaFood Men's One Daily: Offers key vitamins like zinc, vitamin C, and D for men's reproductive health.

Vital Proteins Collagen Peptides: Adds protein and amino acids to support both partners' health and wellness.

The fertility nutrition protocol focuses on nutrient-dense foods, smart supplements, and lifestyle adjustments to prepare your body for pregnancy. By focusing on real, whole foods and essential nutrients, you'll create a strong foundation for conception and overall reproductive health.

Healthy eating for pregnant or breastfeeding women

You only need about 300 extra calories per day to provide sufficient nutrition for your growing baby. However, gaining some weight is natural and necessary during pregnancy, and nursing can help with weight loss after the baby is born. So follow the nutrition protocol, just add in the nutrition tips below to hit optimal pregnancy health.

PROTOCOL FOR PREGNANCY: NOURISHING YOU AND YOUR BABY

Prioritize nutrient-dense foods to support your baby's growth and manage pregnancy symptoms.

Nutrition Tips:

Add Omega-3s: Essential for your baby's brain and visual development. Aim for two servings of cold-water fish weekly (like salmon or sardines). Vegetarian options include seaweed and chia seeds.

High-Quality Proteins: For baby's brain and nervous system, focus on protein from poultry, fish, dairy, and plant sources.

Extra Calories & Small Meals: You only need about 300 extra calories daily, so eat smaller, more frequent meals to help with morning sickness and heartburn.

Avoid Certain Foods: Skip alcohol entirely and limit caffeine. Also, avoid high-mercury fish (like swordfish and albacore tuna), deli meats, raw sprouts, and soft cheeses to reduce the risk of harmful contaminants.

Hacks & Tips:

Snack Smart: Keep easy snacks like yogurt, nuts, and pre-cut veggies on hand to help maintain energy without large meals.

Stay Hydrated: Sipping on water or herbal teas can help ease nausea.

Choose Low-Caffeine Alternatives: Try herbal teas instead of coffee to keep your caffeine intake low.

Brands to Consider:

Nordic Naturals (Omega-3 supplements), **Vital Farms** (pasture-raised eggs), **Organic Valley** (high-quality dairy)

PROTOCOL FOR BREASTFEEDING: BOOSTING NUTRITION FOR MILK PRODUCTION

Maintain a balanced diet to support milk production and energy levels for you and your baby.

Nutrition Tips:

Increase Calories: Nursing moms need slightly more calories—add in an extra healthy snack or two.

Focus on Protein & Calcium: Boost protein by 20 grams daily with sources like Greek yogurt, eggs, nuts, or legumes. Choose calcium-rich foods like leafy greens, broccoli, or dairy to support bone health.

Keep Prenatals Going: Continue taking prenatal vitamins, which help maintain essential nutrients during breastfeeding.

Watch for Allergens: If your baby shows signs of a food sensitivity (e.g., fussiness, skin issues), consider temporarily eliminating common allergens like dairy, eggs, or wheat.

Hacks & Tips:

Hydrate Often: Keep a water bottle handy since breastfeeding increases hydration needs.

Prep Protein-Packed Snacks: Quick options like hard-boiled eggs, cheese, and nut butter keep energy up between meals.

Minimize Caffeine & Alcohol: Try caffeine-free alternatives like herbal tea to stay within safe limits.

Brands to Consider:

Siggi's (high-protein yogurt), **Vital Proteins** (collagen for extra protein), **Traditional Medicinals** (lactation teas for milk support)

These protocols provide simple, actionable steps and tips to support both mom and baby during conception, pregnancy and breastfeeding, focusing on whole foods, nutrient-rich choices, and a few mindful dietary adjustments.

FAQS

Q: Is healthy eating more expensive?

A: It doesn't have to be! Buying in bulk, using pantry staples, and planning meals can help save money. Plus, the money you save on takeout and snack binges adds up.

Q: What if my kids won't eat this stuff?

A: Start small. Add new foods gradually and let them help prep. And remember, you're setting an example—they'll catch on!

Q: Do I need to be 100% organic?

A: Nope! Focus on the Clean 15 and Dirty Dozen for produce. If organic isn't in the budget, rinse produce well, and prioritize whole, minimally processed foods.

Q: What if I mess up and eat something "unhealthy"?
A: No guilt! Enjoy it, move on, and get back to your routine. Healthy eating is about balance, not perfection.

Q: How do I stay motivated?

A: Keep it simple and don't overthink it. Check your energy and mood after a week or two—you'll feel the difference, and that can be the best motivator.

Q: Can I still have treats?

A: Absolutely! Just look for ways to make treats a bit healthier—think dark chocolate, homemade baked goods, or fruit-based desserts.

Q: Is there a quick go-to meal I can make anytime?

A: A grain bowl! Toss cooked grains, a protein, veggies, and a drizzle of sauce. Easy, customizable, and packed with nutrients.

Q: What if I don't have time for meal prep?

A: Opt for easy wins like pre-washed salad greens, frozen veggies, or rotisserie chicken. Small shortcuts make healthy eating more accessible.

Q: How do I get more protein?

A: Add eggs, Greek yogurt, nuts, seeds, beans, or quality meats to meals. Even smoothies can be boosted with a scoop of protein powder.

This protocol isn't about making things harder; it's about setting you up for success with real food that makes you feel awesome. Little by little, these habits will become part of your everyday routine—keeping you nourished, energized, and feeling good in your own skin.

Exercise & Movement: Finding What Works for You

Why This Protocol Matters

Let's be real: You already know exercise is good for you. But between wrangling kids, managing a never-ending to-do list, and keeping everyone alive, finding the time and energy to work out can feel impossible. The good news? You don't need to spend hours at the gym, or follow a complicated fitness plan to get the benefits of movement.

This protocol is about making **exercise work for you**, in a way that feels manageable and energizing, without adding stress to your life. The goal isn't to get a six-pack (unless you want to). It's to feel stronger, more capable, and more in control of your own health.

WHAT TO EXPECT: THE POSSIBILITIES

More Energy: Even short bursts of movement can increase stamina and reduce fatigue.

Better Mood & Less Stress: Exercise is a natural stress reliever and mood booster.

A Stronger, More Resilient Body: Strength training helps with daily tasks like lifting kids and groceries.

Improved Sleep: Exercise supports melatonin production, aiding restful sleep.

Hormone Balance: Movement helps regulate cortisol and support a healthy metabolism.

Reduced Risk of Chronic Disease: Exercise improves heart health, lowers blood pressure, and stabilizes blood sugar.

More Flexibility & Less Pain: Stretching and low-impact exercises prevent stiffness and injury.

A Positive Example for Kids: Showing them that movement is part of a healthy lifestyle.

A Sense of Accomplishment: Completing a short workout is still a win.

A Stronger Mind-Body Connection: Learning to listen to what movement your body needs each day.

Tools & Materials That May Come In Handy

You don't need a gym membership or fancy equipment to get started. A few simple tools can make workouts easier, more effective, and more fun.

Yoga mat for stretching, yoga, or home workouts.

Resistance bands for strength training without heavy weights.

Dumbbells or household items (water bottles, laundry baskets) for strength training.

Supportive sneakers for walking or jogging.

Fitness apps or online videos for quick, guided workouts.

Water bottle to stay hydrated.

Exercise ball for core strengthening and back support.

Jump ropes, mini trampolines, or hula hoops for fun, kid-friendly movement.

These tools make it easier to integrate exercise into your busy life, keeping workouts accessible, fun, and aligned with your goals.

THE CHECKLIST

☐ **Check yourself before you wreck yourself**
Take a moment to assess your current state: Are you running on fumes? Adrenals shot? Chronic pain? If your body's waving a red flag, address those issues first, because the goal here is to feel better, not worse. Start where you are, not where Instagram says you should be.

☐ **Clear the landmines**
Make sure you have a kid-free zone (or at least a semi-kid-safe one) to work out in. Tripping over LEGO bricks mid-squat is not the kind of full-body workout you're aiming for. A yoga mat in the living room works just fine. Bonus if it's not covered in Cheerios.

☐ **Suit Up (but Keep It Real)**
Dig out a pair of leggings that don't cut off circulation and a supportive sports bra that doesn't feel like a medieval torture device. No fancy matching sets required. (Your old band T-shirt totally counts as athleisure.)

☐ **Gather Your Gear (or Improvise)**
No dumbbells? No problem. Raid the pantry for canned goods, grab the kids for resistance (piggyback squats, anyone?), or use your own bodyweight. This isn't about perfection, it's about working with what you've got.

☐ **Set the Mood (and Your Expectations)**
Blast your favorite playlist, grab a water bottle, and remind yourself that some movement is better than no movement. This isn't about crushing a triathlon; it's about taking 10 minutes to remind your body that it's alive and capable. You've got this, mama!

Moving your body improves your mood, boosts your energy, and helps you feel like you again. Whether you're postpartum, deep in toddler chaos, or just trying to keep up with the endless demands of motherhood.

ACTIONABLE STEPS

Movement Quick Guide	
Step 1	Start with Mini Workouts
Step 2	Use What You Have
Step 3	Make Movement Part of Your Day
Step 4	Family Fitness = Less Stress, More Fun

Step 1: Start with Mini Workouts

You don't need an hour-long session to get results. Start with 10-15 minutes of movement, whether it's stretching, a quick strength session, or walking outside.

Try a simple bodyweight circuit:

Squats – 10 reps

Push-ups – 10 reps

Lunges – 10 reps each leg

Plank hold – 30 seconds

Repeat for 2-3 rounds

If you're short on time, sneak in movement throughout the day. Squats while cooking, calf raises while brushing your teeth, or a quick dance session with the kids.

Step 2: Use What You Have

You don't need a gym or fancy equipment. Use your own body weight or get creative with household items.

Use a laundry basket for deadlifts.

Hold a gallon of water for weighted squats.

Do push-ups against a sturdy table if full push-ups feel too intense.

Take the stairs instead of the elevator.

Step 3: Make Movement Part of Your Day

The easiest way to stay consistent is to weave movement into your routine instead of trying to carve out extra time.

Walk while on the phone instead of sitting.

Do squats or lunges while waiting for water to boil.

Stretch before bed instead of scrolling social media.

Take a 10-minute walk after meals to aid digestion and get some fresh air.

Step 4: Family Fitness = Less Stress, More Fun

Getting kids involved turns exercise into playtime rather than a chore.

Dance party in the living room – Pick a song and go all out.

Create a backyard obstacle course – Kids love climbing and jumping.

Race your toddler to the mailbox – They think it's a game, you get your heart rate up.

Do stroller lunges while taking a walk.

EXAMPLE 7 DAY PLAN

Move More, Stress Less, and Feel Stronger—One Small Step at a Time

How It Works:

This plan is designed to fit into your real-life schedule, quick, effective workouts that take 10-20 minutes max. No gym required. No overcomplicated routines. Just movement that works for you.

Each day has a focus: strength, cardio, flexibility, or recovery, so you get variety without burning out. Feel free to swap days, adjust the intensity, or even split workouts into mini-sessions throughout the day.

Day 1	STRENGTH & STABILITY (FULL-BODY RESET)
Goal:	Build strength using your own body weight while improving balance & endurance.
Workout:	(10-15 min)
	Squats - 12 reps Push-ups (knee or full) - 10 reps Lunges (each leg) - 10 reps
	Glute Bridges - 15 reps Plank Hold - 30 seconds
	Repeat 2-3 rounds
	Modify if needed: Hold onto a chair for lunges, do push-ups against a wall, or shorten plank time.
	Make it fun: Play your favorite playlist while doing these. Bonus points if you turn it into a challenge with your kids.
Day 2	QUICK CARDIO & CORE
Goal:	Get your heart rate up and activate your core muscles for better posture & energy.

Workout: (15 min - HIIT Style)

Jumping Jacks or March in Place – 30 seconds
High Knees or Step-Taps – 30 seconds

Standing Oblique Twists – 15 reps per side
Leg Lifts (on mat) – 12 reps

Plank Knee Taps – 10 per side
Rest for 30 seconds, repeat 2-3 rounds

Low-impact option: Step side-to-side instead of jumping, slow down movements, and focus on form.

Boost it: If you have time, go for a 10-minute brisk walk.

Day 3   RECOVERY & FLEXIBILITY (STRETCH IT OUT)

Goal: Loosen tight muscles, increase circulation, and reduce stress.

Workout: (10-15 min Yoga & Stretching)

Child's Pose – 30 seconds
Cat-Cow Stretch – 30 seconds

Downward Dog – 30 seconds
Seated Forward Fold – 30 seconds

Standing Side Stretch – 20 seconds per side
Hip Openers (Butterfly Stretch) – 30 seconds

Savasana (Lie Down & Breathe) – 1-2 minutes

Feeling stiff? Hold stretches longer and breathe deeply into tight areas.

Enhance the vibe: Play soft music or do this right before bed to help with relaxation.

Day 4   STRENGHT & RESISTANCE (UPPER BODY FOCUS)

Goal: Strengthen your arms, shoulders, & back (aka, the muscles needed for lifting kids, groceries, and all the things).

Workout: (10-15 min Strength)

Wall Push-ups or Regular Push-ups – 12 reps
Bent-Over Rows (Use Water Bottles/Dumbbells) – 10 reps

Overhead Press (Household Item as Weight) – 10 reps
Tricep Dips (Using a Sturdy Chair) – 12 reps

Plank Shoulder Taps – 10 per side
Repeat 2-3 rounds

No weights? Use canned goods, laundry detergent, or a resistance band.

Want extra burn? Add 5-10 squats between exercises.

Day 5	CARDIO & LEGS (LOW-IMPACT, HIGH ENERGY)

Goal: Boost energy & endurance while toning the lower body.

Workout: (10-15 min Cardio Focus)

Step-Ups (Use Stairs or a Sturdy Step) – 10 reps per leg
Squat Pulses – 15 reps

Side Lunges – 10 per side
Butt Kicks or Marching in Place – 30 seconds

Calf Raises – 12 reps
Rest 30 seconds, repeat 2-3 rounds

Modify if needed: Use a chair for balance on lunges, slow down, or skip jumps.
On-the-go hack: If you're busy, just walk briskly for 15-20 minutes!

Day 6	FAMILY FUN FITNESS (MAKE IT PLAYFUL)

Goal: Move with your kids or partner in a way that feels fun (because workouts don't have to be boring).

Activity Ideas: Dance Party (Full-Out, No Shame) – 10-15 minutes
Backyard Games (Tag, Jump Rope, Frisbee) – 20 minutes
Stroller Walk + Lunges at the Park – 15 minutes
Mini "Obstacle Course" in Your Living Room – 15 minutes

Got a baby?   Try a "Mommy & Me" Workout—squats while holding them, lunges while pushing the stroller, or baby-wearing marches.

The Goal: Move in *any* way that makes you smile.

Day 7	RESTORE & RESET (STRETCH & SELF-CARE)
Goal:	Ease tension, support recovery, and check in with how your body feels.
Relaxation Routine:	(10-15 min Stretch & Breathe)
	Neck Rolls & Shoulder Shrugs – 30 seconds Seated Spinal Twist – 20 seconds per side
	Hip Flexor Stretch – 30 seconds per side Hamstring Stretch – 30 seconds per leg
	Deep Breathing (Inhale 4 sec, Hold 4 sec, Exhale 4 sec) – 1-2 minutes
Feeling Sore?	Use a foam roller or massage tight areas with a tennis ball.
Post-workout treat:	Make yourself a cup of tea or a nourishing smoothie, you earned it!

Bonus Tips:

Sneak It In: Do calf raises while washing dishes, squats during TV commercials, or lunges on your way to the laundry room.

Track Progress: Use a fitness tracker or app to celebrate every step, squat, or stretch you fit into your day.

Adjust to Your Energy Levels: Feeling tired? Go for a walk or stretch. Feeling energized? Try a quick HIIT session or strength training.

This schedule is designed to fit into even the busiest week, helping you move more, stress less, and feel stronger without overcomplicating things.

BONUS PROTOCOLS: EXERCISE FOR DIFFERENT PHASES OF MOTHERHOOD

Safe Exercises for Mom and Baby: Move Smart, Feel Strong

Moving your body during pregnancy is not only safe—it's actually encouraged by, oh, everyone. **The World Health Organization**, the **U.S. Department of Health & Human Services,** and **the American College of Obstetrics and Gynecology** all recommend about 150 minutes of moderate exercise a week, ideally spread over at least three days. This is about training your body for something similar to an extreme athletic event. My husband has run over 20 Iron Mans, and when people ask if I train for them too-I say I completed 3-note the three kids standing next to me! Yes-I'm getting real here. Having a baby is equally (if not more challenging-physically and mentally) than completing an Iron Man (and you can quote me on that!) You want to be healthy and strong for this event.

What You Can Do

Here are some mom-and-baby-friendly moves that keep it safe and effective:

Kegels

Oh yes, the unsung hero of pregnancy workouts. Strengthen those pelvic muscles now to help prevent "oops moments" (aka urinary incontinence) later. Bonus: they're discreet. No one will know you're doing them at the dinner table.

Resistance and Strength Training (2 Days a Week)

Build up those larger muscle groups—you're going to need

them for all the baby-hauling ahead. Use light weights, resistance bands, or even just your body weight. Keep it moderate and controlled.

Low-Impact Cardio

Start slow and stick with activities that feel comfortable: **Elliptical Machine**: Smooth and joint-friendly. **Stationary Cycling**: Great for cardio without the wobble risk. **Walking**: The easiest way to get moving—no equipment needed.

Prenatal Yoga

Stretch, strengthen, and zen out while focusing on breathing techniques that might come in handy during labor. I loved these classes-plus I was blessed to have a true Doula as my instructor!

Swimming or Water Aerobics

Water is magical—it takes the weight off your joints, keeps you cool, and gives you a great full-body workout.

WHAT TO SKIP (FOR NOW)

Not all exercises are pregnancy-friendly. Here's what to avoid for you and your babies safety):

1. High-Risk Activities:

- ▶ Anything with a high fall risk (horseback riding and road cycling).

- ▶ Sports with contact or collisions like basketball, soccer, or anything where you're dodging balls and bodies.

2. High-Altitude and Scuba Diving:

- ▶ Nope and nope. These activities can mess with oxygen levels and aren't worth the risk.

3. Overly Rigorous Moves:

- ▶ Skip exercises that require lying flat on your back after the first trimester, as they can restrict blood flow.

- ▶ Avoid activities that feel like too much strain on your abdomen.

Keep Your Cool (Literally)

Pregnancy means your body's working overtime, and regulating your core temperature is one of the things it does differently. The good news? Moderate exercise won't overheat you, as long as you take some basic precautions.

Hot Weather Tips:

- ▶ Plan workouts for early morning or evening when it's cooler.

- ▶ Stay hydrated (always have water within arm's reach).

- ▶ Wear loose, breathable clothing to help your body stay cool.

Cold Weather Tips:

- ▶ Dress in layers, so you can peel off as you warm up.

- ▶ Schedule outdoor activities for midday when it's warmest.

- ▶ If you feel lightheaded or overly fatigued, take a break—your body's already working hard enough growing a tiny human.

Bottom Line

Exercise during pregnancy isn't about pushing your limits—it's about feeling good, staying healthy, and preparing your body for the beautiful chaos that lies ahead of you. Start slow, listen to your body, and don't forget to celebrate the fact that you're moving, because even small steps count in a big way.

FAQS

Q: Can I exercise if I'm trying to conceive?

Answer: Absolutely! Exercise can improve circulation, regulate hormones, and reduce stress, all of which support fertility. Focus on moderate, low-impact workouts like walking, yoga, or light strength training. Just avoid over-training—it can mess with your hormones, especially if you're already dealing with irregular cycles.

Q: Is it safe to work out during pregnancy?

Answer: Yes, as long as you're cleared by your doctor! Stick to moderate-intensity exercises like walking, swimming, or prenatal yoga. Avoid activities with a high risk of falling or heavy impact-sorry skiing and horseback riding! And always listen to your body—if it says "slow down," do it.

Q: What's the best type of exercise during pregnancy?

Answer: The best exercise is the one that feels good and is safe for your body. Walking, swimming, and prenatal yoga are all mom-favorites. Strength training with light weights is great too—just avoid anything that strains your core or requires lying on your back after the first trimester.

Q: How soon can I exercise postpartum?

Answer: It depends on your delivery and recovery. Vaginal births typically allow light movement like walking within a few weeks, while C-section moms may need more time. Wait for your doctor's green light (usually at the 6-week checkup) before starting anything more intense. Start slow—your body's been through a lot!

Q: What exercises are safe postpartum?

Answer: Focus on gentle movements that strengthen your core and pelvic floor, like Kegels, bridges, and light yoga. Avoid heavy lifting and intense cardio until your body feels ready. Diastasis recti (ab separation) is common postpartum, so consult a professional before doing planks or crunches.

Q: I'm 2+ years postpartum—how do I get back into fitness?

Answer: Start with low-impact, consistent movement like walking or yoga, then build up to strength training and cardio. The key is to listen to your body and avoid overdoing it if you're still feeling effects like joint instability or pelvic floor issues. Even years postpartum, it's okay to ease in.

Q: Can I lift weights while pregnant or postpartum?

Answer: Yes, but with caution. During pregnancy, stick to lighter weights to avoid straining your core or back. Postpartum, start slow and focus on core stability before increasing weights. If you have diastasis recti or pelvic floor concerns, consult a trainer or physical therapist first.

Q: How do I make time for exercise as a busy mom?

Answer: Squeeze in 10-15 minutes wherever you can— while the baby naps, during screen time, or even while cooking dinner (hello, counter push-ups!). Movement doesn't have to be all or nothing—dance with your kids, walk while on a call, or do lunges between laundry loads.

Q: What if I'm too tired to work out?

Answer: It's okay! Sleep-deprived moms don't need a

lecture about "pushing through." Start small: a 5-minute walk, some gentle stretches, or even deep breathing counts. Sometimes, a little movement can energize you, but if you're completely wiped out, rest is the best medicine.

Q: How do I know if I'm overdoing it?

Answer: If you feel exhausted, overly sore, lightheaded, or like your workout is making you more stressed, it's time to pull back. Pain (especially in your pelvis, back, or abdomen), leaking, or feeling overly fatigued are signs to slow down or consult a professional. Exercise should feel good, not like punishment!

Sleep for Moms Who Don't Have Time for BS

WHY THIS PROTOCOL MATTERS

Sleep is the real MVP of motherhood, but let's be honest, moms are chronically sleep-deprived. Whether it's pregnancy discomfort, midnight feedings, toddler nightmares, or your brain running through the *1,000 things you forgot to do today*, sleep always seems to get the short end of the stick.

The good news? This protocol isn't about "perfect" sleep. It's about realistic, achievable changes that help you get better rest, even in the middle of the chaos.

What to Expect: The Possibilities

Better Mood & Less Stress: Because snapping at your family isn't fun for anyone.

Balanced Hormones & Fewer Late-Night Cravings: Sleep

regulates hunger and stress hormones, making it easier to say no to that midnight cookie binge.

Sharper Focus & Fewer "Where Did I Put My Keys?" Moments: Because mental fog is so last season.

Stronger Immune System: Moms don't get sick days, so let's keep those germs away.

More Energy (Without Relying on Coffee Alone): Imagine waking up actually feeling refreshed.

Tools & Materials That May Come In Handy

A few simple sleep upgrades can make a world of difference.

Blackout Curtains or Eye Mask: Blocks out light so your brain knows it's bedtime.

White Noise Machine or App: Drowns out snoring partners, noisy neighbors, and that one kid who insists on waking up at 3 AM.

Aromatherapy Diffuser & Oils: Lavender and chamomile help cue your brain to wind down.

Weighted Blanket: Like a hug for your nervous system, reducing anxiety and improving deep sleep.

Comfortable Bedding: Soft, breathable sheets and a supportive pillow = game changer.

Magnesium Supplement: Supports relaxation and sleep quality (check with your doctor first).

Blue Light Blocking Glasses: Helps counteract screen-related sleep disruptions.

Sleep Tracker: Monitors sleep patterns and helps you tweak your routine for better rest.

Calming Teas: Chamomile, valerian root, or a magnesium-rich bedtime drink can work wonders.

Recommended Tools

Apps: Calm, Insight Timer, and Sleep Cycle.

Books: *Why We Sleep* by Matthew Walker, *The Sleep Solution* by W. Chris Winter.

Charts: Sleep hygiene checklists and circadian rhythm planners.

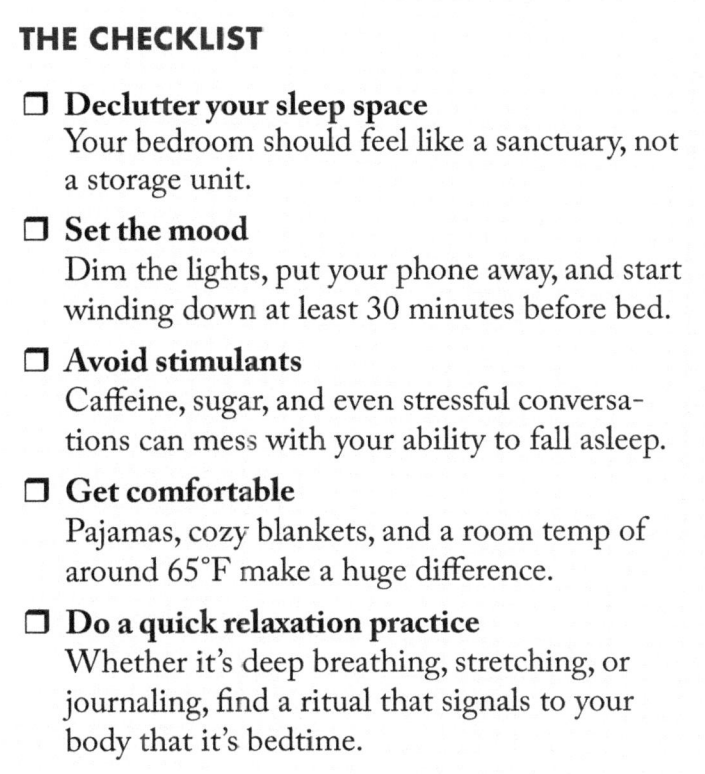

THE CHECKLIST

☐ **Declutter your sleep space**
Your bedroom should feel like a sanctuary, not a storage unit.

☐ **Set the mood**
Dim the lights, put your phone away, and start winding down at least 30 minutes before bed.

☐ **Avoid stimulants**
Caffeine, sugar, and even stressful conversations can mess with your ability to fall asleep.

☐ **Get comfortable**
Pajamas, cozy blankets, and a room temp of around 65°F make a huge difference.

☐ **Do a quick relaxation practice**
Whether it's deep breathing, stretching, or journaling, find a ritual that signals to your body that it's bedtime.

Good sleep equals more patience, fewer meltdowns (yours and theirs), balanced hormones, stronger immunity, and better focus. In short, it's the difference between surviving and *thriving*.

ACTIONALBLE STEPS

Step 1	Create a Sleep Sanctuary
Step 2	Establish a Sleep Routine
Step 3	Limit Screen Time
Step 4	Optimize Nutrition for Sleep
Step 5	Experiment with Natural Sleep Aids
Step 6	Sync with Your Circadian Rhythm
Step 7	Address Underlying Sleep Issues

HERE'S THE BREAKDOWN:

Step 1: Create a Sleep Sanctuary

Your bedroom should be designed for sleep, not stress.

Declutter: No laundry piles, work papers, or bright overhead lights.

Keep it Cool: The ideal sleeping temp is around 65°F.

Block Out Light & Noise: Use blackout curtains, an eye mask, and a white noise machine if needed.

Invest in Good Bedding: Breathable sheets, a supportive pillow, and a comfy mattress make a difference.

Quick Fix: If your sleep space isn't restful, start by making one small improvement—switching out bright lights for warm-toned lamps is an easy first step.

Step 2: Establish a Sleep Routine

Consistency is key. Try to go to bed and wake up at the same time every day, even on weekends.

Start winding down 30-60 minutes before bed.

Incorporate a calming ritual—a warm bath, reading, journaling, or light stretching.

No social media scrolling! Your brain doesn't need late-night drama from the internet.

Hack: Set a "bedtime alarm" as a reminder to start your wind-down routine.

Step 3: Limit Screen Time

Blue light from screens messes with melatonin production, making it harder to fall asleep.

Turn off screens 30-60 minutes before bed.

If you must use your phone, wear blue light-blocking glasses or use night mode.

Replace scrolling with something relaxing—reading, meditation, or a sleep podcast.

Hack: Plug your phone in across the room to resist the temptation of late-night doom-scrolling.

Step 4: Optimize Nutrition for Sleep

What you eat affects how you sleep.

Avoid heavy meals before bed. Your digestive system needs time to rest, too.

Steer clear of caffeine after 2 PM. Even if you think you're not sensitive, you are.

Choose sleep-friendly snacks if needed—bananas, almonds, or chamomile tea.

Hack: Keep a bottle of magnesium spray by your bed—it helps relax muscles and ease you into sleep.

Step 5: Experiment with Natural Sleep Aids
Natural remedies can help queue your body that it's time to sleep.

Magnesium supplements: Supports relaxation and sleep quality.

Aromatherapy: Lavender and chamomile scents help signal bedtime.

Weighted blankets: Helps calm the nervous system and reduce anxiety.

Hack: Try the 4-7-8 breathing technique before bed: inhale for 4 seconds, hold for 7, exhale for 8.

Step 6: Sync with Your Circadian Rhythm
Your body has a built-in clock—work with it, not against it.

Get morning sunlight within an hour of waking up.

Dim lights in the evening to mimic natural sunset queues.

Stick to a routine—your body thrives on consistency.

Hack: If you wake up feeling groggy, get outside for 10 minutes of sunlight—it helps reset your internal clock.

Step 7: Address Underlying Sleep Issues

If sleep problems persist, don't ignore them.

Keep a sleep journal to track patterns and identify triggers.

Talk to a doctor if you experience chronic insomnia, snoring, or sleep apnea symptoms.

Adjust lifestyle factors—stress, hormones, and nutrition all play a role.

Hack: Use a sleep tracker (like **Oura Ring or Fitbit**) to monitor trends and make adjustments.

EXAMPLE 7 DAY PLAN

Because You Deserve More Than Just a Few
Hours of Broken Sleep

This one-week sleep reset is designed to help you build better habits, reclaim your rest, and wake up feeling *less like a zombie and more like a functioning human*. Each day focuses on one small, manageable step—because let's be real, overhauling your sleep in one night is impossible (especially if you have kids waking up at random hours).

How to Use This Plan:

Follow each day's action step and build on it throughout the week.

Adjust based on your schedule, energy levels, and sleep struggles.

Progress, not perfection—if you miss a step, just get back on track the next day.

Day 1	DECLUTTER & SET UP YOUR SLEEP SANCTUARY
	Your bedroom should be a peaceful escape, not an extension of your to-do list.
Action:	Remove laundry piles, work papers, and random clutter.
	Dim the lights and set up blackout curtains or an eye mask.
	Keep the room cool (around 65°F) for optimal sleep.
Why?	A clean, cozy space signals to your brain that your bedroom equals rest, not stress.

Day 2	SET A SLEEP SCHEDULE (YES, EVEN FOR MOMS)
	Your body craves routine, let's give it one.
Action:	Pick a bedtime and wake-up time that you can (mostly) stick to.
	Adjust in small increments if needed (start with 15-30 min earlier or later).
	Try to wake up at the same time daily, even on weekends.
Why?	A consistent schedule helps reset your internal clock and makes falling asleep easier.

Day 3	CREATE A WIND-DOWN ROUTINE
	Bedtime isn't just for kids, you need a routine, too.
Action:	Choose a pre-bed ritual (warm bath, reading, light stretching, or journaling).
	Dim the lights 30-60 minutes before bed.
	Cut back on stimulating activities—no intense workouts or late-night doom-scrolling.
Why?	A consistent pre-sleep ritual signals your body that it's time to shut down.

Day 4	LIMIT SCREEN TIME BEFORE BED
	Blue light s a melatonin killer.
Action:	Turn off screens 30-60 minutes before bed.
	If you must use screens, switch to night mode or wear blue light-blocking glasses.
	Charge your phone outside your bedroom (or across the room).
Why?	Blue light disrupts melatonin production, making it harder to fall asleep.

Day 5	TRY AROMATHERAPY OR A CALMING TEA
	Because your nervous system deserves a little love.
Action:	Diffuse lavender essential oil or use a pillow spray.
	Sip on chamomile or valerian root tea 30-45 minutes before bed.
	Try a magnesium supplement (check with your doctor first).
Why?	Certain scents and teas help relax your body and mind, making it easier to drift off.

Day 6	ADD GENTLE MOVEMENT TO YOUR NIGHT ROUTINE
	Shake off the stress of the day, without overdoing it.
Action:	Do 10 minutes of gentle stretching, yoga, or deep breathing.
	Try legs-up-the-wall pose for 5 minutes, it's magic for calming the nervous system.
	Avoid intense exercise too close to bedtime.
Why?	Gentle movement releases tension and preps your body for deep rest.

Day 7	REFLECT & FINE-TUNE YOUR SLEEP PLAN
	What's working? What's not? Adjust as needed.
Action:	Review what helped you sleep best this week.
	Keep a sleep journal for a few nights: track bedtime, wake time, and sleep quality.
	Adjust anything that isn't working (timing, routines, bedroom setup).
Why?	Tracking progress helps you see patterns and make adjustments for long-term success

BONUS TIPS FOR BETTER SLEEP

If You Struggle to Fall Asleep:

Try the 4-7-8 breathing technique (inhale for 4 sec, hold for 7, exhale for 8).

Listen to a sleep meditation or calming sounds.

Keep a notepad by your bed for late-night thoughts that keep you awake.

If You Wake Up in the Middle of the Night:

Avoid checking your phone (no doom-scrolling!).

Get up, stretch, or do deep breathing if needed, don't force sleep.

Keep lights dim if you have to move around.

If You're Exhausted During the Day:

Get morning sunlight within an hour of waking up. It helps regulate your body clock.

230

Take a 10-20 minute nap if needed (but avoid long naps late in the day).

Stay hydrated. Sometimes fatigue is just dehydration in disguise.

FAQ'S

Q. How many hours of sleep do moms really need?

A. Aim for 7-9 hours, but quality matters more than quantity. The point is to wake up feeling refreshed, not disheveled.

Q. What's the best bedtime for moms?

A. Between 9-10 P.M is ideal for syncing with natural circadian rhythms. Moon goes up-Mom goes to bed.

Q. Can I nap during the day?

A. Yes, but keep it to 20-30 minutes to avoid nighttime disruptions. You are one of the lucky ones if you can. So just do it!

Q. How do I get better sleep postpartum?

A. Sleep when the baby sleeps (I know this one is easier said than done, but it is the best way to catch up on some zzz's), and create a supportive sleep routine with your partner-they are fully capable to get up and do bottle feedings and diaper changes. Just ask.

Q. Can hormones really mess with my sleep?

A. Absolutely. Hormonal fluctuations can disrupt your rest—talk to your doctor if it's an ongoing issue. You may need to take supplements or perhaps you're not taking the proper dose.

Q. Do weighted blankets actually work?

A. Many moms swear by them for reducing anxiety and promoting deeper sleep. It's like having a force pinning you in bed. Oh wait, that's exactly what it is!

Q. Is screen time really that bad for sleep?

A. Yes, blue light can interfere with melatonin production, making it harder to fall asleep. (Cue hormone disruption!)

Q. What's the best snack before bed?

A. A banana or pistachios are great options—they're light and promote sleep. But, always try to stop eating two hours before bed time.

Q. Can exercise improve my sleep?

A. Definitely! Just avoid high-intensity workouts too close to bedtime. Don't get the adrenaline pumping before you close your eyes. Try out restorative yoga or tai chi.

Q. When should I see a doctor about sleep issues?

A. If you're consistently struggling with sleep despite making changes, it's time to consult a healthcare provider. You should not feel like a zombie, or as if you're floating through your day in a bubble. It doesn't mean you are doing anything wrong. Birth is taxing on a body-and that can last for years. So many things can disrupt our sleep from hormone disruption to food. I tend to lean towards a functional doctor to find the root cause, but go to the doctor you can, and demand to discover the cause.

Sleep isn't just about feeling less cranky (though that's a huge bonus). **It's a lifeline** for your mental health. Chronic sleep deprivation can skyrocket your stress, ramp up anxiety, and drag you into the murky waters of depression. And let's be real, moms are pros at putting everyone else first, often at the expense of their own well-being.

Mindset & Mental Health for Moms

WHY THIS PROTOCOL MATTERS

Motherhood is basically running a full-time business, except your employees don't listen, your office is always messy, and there's no PTO. If your brain feels like a browser with 50 tabs open, and you can't figure out which one is playing music, you're not alone.

Your mental health affects everything. Your mood, energy, parenting style, patience level, and how you handle the daily chaos. And while you can't eliminate stress *(because, kids)*, you can manage it in a way that keeps you from completely losing your mind.

This protocol isn't about becoming some "zen goddess" who never gets overwhelmed *(seriously, that's not a thing)*. It's about practical, realistic ways to shift your mindset, reduce stress, and create mental space so you can actually enjoy life, without waiting until your kids are grown.

What To Expect: The Possibilities

Less Stress & Overwhelm: Say goodbye to full-blown mental spirals and hello to small, simple ways to keep your cool.

A Better Mood (with Less Mom Guilt): Fewer rage-y moments, more laugh-y ones.

Improved Sleep: No more 3 a.m. overthinking marathons.

More Patience: Because tantrums, sibling fights, and "Mom! Mom! Mom!" on repeat require next-level emotional endurance.

Stronger Relationships: Less resentment, more connection (with your kids, partner, and yourself).

More Energy (Without Surviving on Just Coffee & Sheer Willpower): Because mental exhaustion is just as draining as physical exhaustion.

Tools & Materials That May Come In Handy

A few simple tools can help shift your mindset and reduce daily stress—without requiring hours of effort.

Gratitude Journal: Helps you focus on the good (even if it's just, "I drank my coffee while it was still hot!").

Mindfulness Apps: Quick, guided meditations for those "I might snap" moments.

Cozy Chair or Meditation Cushion: For your designated "calm corner" in the house.

Foam Roller or Yoga Mat: Quick tension relief for when

stress starts creeping into your muscles.

Noise-Canceling Headphones: Because sometimes, you just need silence.

Aromatherapy Diffuser & Essential Oils: Lavender, chamomile, and citrus scents can help bring a little calm to the chaos.

Boundaries Workbook: Because learning to say "no" without guilt is a superpower.

Brain-Boosting Snacks: You can't regulate emotions when you're hangry.

A Timer or Reminder App: To make sure you actually take breaks.

Support System Tools: Whether it's a group chat, an online community, or just one friend who gets it.

Recommended Tools and Resources

Books: *Burnout* by Emily Nagoski, *The Happiness* Project by Gretchen Rubin.

Apps: Calm, Insight Timer, Forest for focus.

Workbooks: *The Anti-Anxiety Notebook*, *How to Do the Work* by Dr. Nicole LePera.

Podcasts: *The Life Coach School, The Mom Hour.*

THE CHECKLIST

☐ **Find 10 minutes a day**
That's it. If you can scroll Instagram, you can do this.

☐ **Set up a mindfulness corner**
A chair, a journal, maybe a diffuser—just a small, calming space.

☐ **Pick one task to delegate this week**
Yes, it's okay to ask for help.

☐ **Make a list of energy drains**
Identify 3 things that exhaust you and set one boundary around them.

☐ **Commit to baby steps**
No perfection required. One small habit at a time = long-term change.

Don't feel like you have to cram all these in within one or or one week even, or feel like you HAVE to do all of these. If even just one stands out to you, try it out for one week and see if that helps! Then add another the week following. It never hurts to try anything once. The best part, no one will know, except you!

ACTIONABLE STEPS

QUCK GUIDE	
Step 1	Morning Mindfulness
Step 2	Take Active Breaks
Step 3	Practice Gratitude
Step 4	Set Boundaries
Step 5	Strengthen Relationships
Step 6	Eat for Mental Clarity

Step 1: Morning Mindfulness (Start Your Day on Your Terms)

Your first **5-10 minutes set the tone** for the entire day.

Action:

Do **5-10 minutes of mindfulness**—deep breathing, meditation, or just drinking coffee in peace.

Try a breathing exercise—inhale for 4 seconds, hold for 4, exhale for 4.

Use a morning mantra—something simple like "I can handle whatever today brings."

Think of one thing you're grateful for before checking your phone.

Why?

Starting the day **calmly and intentionally** helps you feel *in control* instead of *reactive*.

Step 2: Take Active Breaks
(Move to Reset Your Mind)

When stress builds up, **move your body to release it**.

Action:

Take **2-minute active breaks** throughout the day: stretch, walk, dance, shake it out.

Set a **reminder** to stand up and move every hour.

Do a "tension check"—if your shoulders are up by your ears, it's time to stretch.

Why?

Physical movement helps **reset your nervous system**, preventing stress from building up.

Step 3: Practice Gratitude
(Train Your Brain to See the Good)

Gratitude isn't just a *feel-good* thing—it **literally rewires your brain** to focus on the positives.

Action:

Write **three things you're grateful for** every night *(even if it's just "I survived today")*.

Share **one gratitude moment** at dinner with your family.

Try a **gratitude jar**—write small wins and read them back at the end of the month.

Why?

Your brain is wired to focus on problems—**gratitude helps balance the negativity bias**.

Step 4: Set Boundaries (Because You Can't Do It All)

Protect your time, energy, and **sanity**.

Action:

Say "no" when needed—without guilt.

Delegate one thing this week—chores, work, mental load tasks.

Limit digital distractions—turn off notifications, unfollow stress-inducing accounts.

Schedule "me time" daily—even if it's just 10 minutes alone.

Why?

Overcommitting = burnout. Setting limits gives you mental space to *breathe*.

Step 5: Strengthen Relationships (Because We're Not Meant to Do This Alone)

Action:

Call or text **one supportive friend** today.

Plan a **weekly check-in** with someone who lifts you up.

Set limits on toxic relationships (less time, fewer interactions, stronger boundaries).

Join an **online or in-person moms' group** for support.

Why?

Connection reduces stress, increases happiness, and helps you feel less alone.

Step 6: Eat for Mental Clarity (Fuel Your Brain Right)

What you eat directly affects your mood and stress levels.

Action:

Eat **more omega-3s** (salmon, walnuts, chia seeds).

Add **magnesium-rich foods** (almonds, spinach, dark chocolate).

Reduce sugar crashes by choosing whole foods over processed junk.

Keep **healthy snacks nearby**—because hanger is real.

Why?

Balanced blood sugar = **fewer mood swings, more mental clarity.**

EXAMPLE 7 DAY PLAN

Reduce Stress, Shift Your Mindset, and Feel More Like Yourself Again

Motherhood is non-stop, and mental overload is *real*. This 7-day plan is designed to help you reduce stress, set boundaries, and create space for yourself—without adding more to your plate. Each day builds on the last, so by the end of the week, you'll have small, sustainable habits that make a big impact on your mental well-being.

How to Use This Plan:

Follow each day's simple action step (most take 10 minutes or less!).

If a day doesn't go as planned, just pick up where you left off—progress over perfection.

Adjust based on what feels right for your energy, stress levels, and needs.

Day 1	**FIND 10 MINUTES FOR YOURSELF (YES, YOU HAVE TIME!)**
	Start small—carve out a few intentional minutes just for YOU.
Action:	Block out **10 minutes** for a mindful moment—deep breathing, journaling, or sitting quietly with your coffee (without distractions).
	Set a reminder on your phone if needed.
	Tell your family: "This is my 10 minutes. I'll be back." (They will survive.)
Why?	Taking **even a few minutes daily** helps **reduce stress, increase focus, and give your brain a break.**

Day 2	**CREATE A MINDFULNESS CORNER**
	Make a space in your home that reminds you to pause and reset.
Action:	Find a **small space** for your "calm corner" (a chair, a cushion, a spot in your bedroom).
	Add **one calming element**—a journal, essential oils, a cozy blanket.
	Use this space **once today**, even if it's just for **one deep breath**.
Why?	Having a physical reminder to pause helps make mindfulness a habit, not an afterthought.

Day 3	**DOWNLOAD A MINDFULNESS OR BREATHING APP**
	Let technology work for you instead of stressing you out.
Action:	Download an app like **Calm, Insight Timer, or Headspace**.
	Try **one 5-minute meditation today**—either guided or just deep breathing.
	Don't overthink it—press play, listen, and breathe.
Why?	Apps **make mindfulness easy** by guiding you through simple exercises, even when your brain feels overloaded.

Day 4	DELEGATE ONE TASK (BECAUSE YOU CAN'T DO IT ALL)
	Lighten your mental load—ask for help (without guilt!)
Action:	Pick **one thing to delegate**—dishes, laundry, bedtime routine, grocery pickup.
	Tell your partner, kids, or a friend: "I need a little help with this."
	Resist the urge to redo it *(perfectionism is not your friend here!)*.
Why?	Sharing responsibilities **reduces stress and prevents burnout**—plus, it teaches your family that **mom is not a one-woman show**.

Day 5	SET A BOUNDARY AROUND ENERGY DRAINS
	Protect your time, energy, and sanity.
Action:	List **three things that drain you** (constant notifications, toxic conversations, overcommitting).
	Choose **one boundary** to implement today—turn off notifications, say no to something, set a time limit for social media.
	Stick to it—remind yourself that **protecting your energy is not selfish**.
Why?	Setting boundaries **reduces overwhelm and helps you focus on what truly matters**.

Day 6	CONNECT WITH SOMEONE WHO LIFTS YOU UP
	You're not meant to do this alone—find your people.
Action:	Call, text, or voice message one supportive friend today.
	If you're feeling isolated, join an online or in-person moms' group.

Schedule a quick coffee date or a phone call (even 5 minutes counts).

| Why? | Social connection **reduces stress, improves mood, and reminds you that you're not alone**. |

| **Day 7** | **START A GRATITUDE PRACTICE** |

Shift your mindset by focusing on what's good—even in the chaos.

| Action: | Write down **3 things you're grateful for today**. |

Make this a **nightly habit**—before bed, jot down **small wins** (hot coffee, toddler snuggles, a quiet moment).

Keep a **Gratitude Jar**—write daily gratitudes on paper and read them at the end of the month.

| Why? | Gratitude **literally rewires your brain** to focus on the pos - tives, reducing stress and increasing resilience. |

SMALL SHIFTS = BIG CHANGES

Mental health isn't about having it all together. It's about making small, sustainable changes that help you feel more calm, present, and in control.

Even 10 minutes a day can help you reset, refocus, and build the resilience to handle whatever motherhood throws at you.

So start today, one small step, one mindset shift, one moment at a time.

Because you deserve peace too.

BONUS TIPS FOR AN ONGOING MENTAL HEALTH RESET

If You're Feeling Overwhelmed:

Take 5 deep breaths—inhale for 4, hold for 4, exhale for 4.

Do a 10-minute walk outside—fresh air = instant mental clarity.

Put your phone away for an hour—reduce digital clutter.

If You're Feeling Drained:

Drink a glass of water—dehydration worsens brain fog.

Eat a brain-boosting snack—almonds, dark chocolate, Greek yogurt.

Take a power nap—20 minutes max, no guilt.

If You're Struggling with Mom Guilt:

Remind yourself: "I don't have to be perfect to be a great mom."

Delegate without guilt—sharing responsibilities benefits everyone.

Do one thing for yourself daily—happy moms raise happy kids.

FAQ'S

Q: How do I find time for self-care with a packed schedule?

Answer: Start small. Even 5 minutes of mindfulness or stretching counts. Consistency matters more than length.

Q: What if I feel guilty taking time for myself?

Answer: Remember, taking care of yourself helps you take better care of your family. You can't pour from an empty cup.

Q: How do I stop overthinking everything?

Answer: Use grounding techniques like the 5-4-3-2-1

method (identify 5 things you see, 4 you feel, etc.) to pull yourself out of overthinking mode.

Q: Can this really reduce my stress?

Answer: Yes! Small, consistent changes, like gratitude journaling and active breaks, can significantly reduce stress over time.

Q: What's the best app for quick mindfulness?

Answer: Headspace and Calm are great for guided meditations under 10 minutes.

Q: How do I set boundaries without feeling like a bad mom?

Answer: Focus on your priorities. Saying "no" to one thing is saying "yes" to what really matters.

Q: Why is gratitude so important?

Answer: It shifts your focus from what's stressful to what's good, boosting your mood and perspective.

Q: What if my partner isn't supportive?

Answer: Share why this matters to you and invite them to join in small ways, like a gratitude practice or active breaks together.

Q: How long before I see results?

Answer: You might notice small changes in a few days, but real, lasting results come with consistency over weeks.

Q: Can I still benefit if I don't do every step?

Answer: Absolutely. Start with one or two steps and build from there. Progress is what counts, not perfection.

Natural Beauty Care

*Ditch the Toxins, Simplify Your Routine,
and Let Your Natural Glow Shine*

WHY THIS PROTOCOL MATTERS

Beauty products today are a toxic minefield—loaded with chemicals, artificial fragrances, and endocrine disruptors that do more harm than good. And let's not even get started on the pressure to chase "perfection" with Botox, fillers, and endless anti-aging serums. The truth? Wrinkles won't kill you, but chronic inflammation from foreign substances might.

This Natural Beauty Care Protocol is about simplifying your routine, swapping harmful products for safe, effective, and natural alternatives, and embracing real, healthy skin—without the constant battle against aging.

What To Expect: The Possibilities

Glowing Skin – Hydration, nourishment, and real, natural radiance.

249

Reduced Chemical Exposure: Fewer endocrine disruptors, more peace of mind.

Simplified Routine: No more cluttered cabinets full of half-used products.

Cost Savings: Natural beauty is often cheaper than over-priced, chemical-heavy creams.

Sustainability: Many natural alternatives are eco-friendly and planet-conscious.

Customizable Skincare: No one-size-fits-all products—just tailored care for your skin type.

Confidence Boost: Because knowing your skincare is nourishing rather than harming is empowering.

Tools & Materials That May Come In Handy

A few simple swaps make a huge difference for your skin's health.

Hydration Tools: Large water bottle + electrolytes to support glowing skin from within.

Natural Oils: Coconut oil, jojoba oil, shea butter for hydration and cleansing.

DIY Face Mask Ingredients: Honey, oats, avocado, yogurt for easy, effective treatments.

Humidifier: Helps prevent dry skin (especially in colder months).

Wooden Comb: Gentle on hair, prevents breakage, and distributes natural oils.

Witch Hazel: A natural toner for balancing and refreshing the skin.

Reusable Cotton Rounds: Eco-friendly and gentler than

disposable wipes.

Blue Light Blocking Glasses: Protects skin from screen-induced premature aging.

Clean Pillowcases & Bedding: Your skin rests on them all night—keep them soft, breathable, and toxin-free.

Apps to Help You Detox Your Beauty Routine:

Think Dirty App: Scan product barcodes for ingredient safety ratings.

Yuka App: Instantly see if your products contain harmful chemicals.

EWG Skin Deep Database: Research clean, non-toxic beauty products.

THE CHECKLIST

❐ **Audit your current products**
Use the Yuka App or Think Dirty to check for harmful ingredients.

❐ **Hydrate like it's your job**
Drink ½ your body weight in ounces of water daily for better skin.

❐ **Stock up on natural beauty essentials**
Coconut oil, aloe vera, witch hazel, and hydrating face mists.

❐ **Clean your beauty tools**
Wash makeup brushes regularly (bacteria buildup = breakouts).

❐ **Create a simple beauty schedule**
Swap one product at a time and track how your skin responds.

No need to throw everything out at once—replace as you go, make small changes, and create a beauty routine that supports your skin and overall health.

Because beauty isn't about looking airbrushed. It's about taking care of yourself—naturally, sustainably, and without hidden toxins sabotaging your glow.

ACTIONABLE STEPS

QUICK GUIDE	
Step 1	Hydrate Inside and Out
Step 2	Detox Your Skincare Routine
Step 3	Try a DIY Face Mask
Step 4	Switch to Oil Cleansing
Step 5	Add a Hydrating Mist
Step 6	Deep Condition Your Hair Naturally
Step 7	Track Progress & Plan Your Next Swaps

Step 1: Hydrate Inside and Out

Action:

Drink ½ your body weight in ounces of water daily.

Apply coconut oil or shea butter post-shower for deep hydration.

Tips & Hacks:

Set a water-tracking goal using an app.

Add electrolytes or a squeeze of lemon for better absorption.

Apply coconut oil while skin is still damp for better penetration.

Favorite Products:

Stanley or Hydro Flask water bottles.

Ultima Replenisher Electrolytes.

Step 2: Detox Your Skincare Routine
Action:

Toss expired or chemical-heavy products (use the **Yuka App**—anything under 75 should go!).

Swap to 3–5 core products that actually nourish your skin.

Tips & Hacks:

Read ingredients—if you can't pronounce it, your skin probably doesn't need it.

Ditch fragrance & dyes—common irritants that do more harm than good.

Start with ONE swap at a time to avoid overwhelming your skin.

Favorite Apps:
Think Dirty App

EWG's Skin Deep Database

Step 3: Try a DIY Face Mask
Action:

Mix honey + yogurt for hydration and gentle exfoliation.

Tips & Hacks:

Add turmeric for anti-inflammatory benefits.

Apply while multitasking—fold laundry, sip tea, or relax.

Favorite Ingredients:

Manuka Honey

Organic Turmeric Powder

Step 4: Switch to Oil Cleansing
Action:

Swap soap-based cleansers for oil cleansing (jojoba or squalane oil).

Tips & Hacks:

Double cleanse if wearing makeup (oil first, then rinse with a warm cloth).

For acne-prone skin, add a drop of tea tree oil.

For dry skin, mix in argan oil.

Favorite Oils:

Cliganic Organic Jojoba Oil

The Ordinary Squalane Cleanser

Step 5: Add a Hydrating Mist
Action:

Use rosewater mist midday for a refreshing glow.

Tips & Hacks:

DIY your mist—mix rosewater with aloe vera.

Keep it in the fridge for a cooling effect.

Favorite Products:

Heritage Store Rosewater

Cocokind Rosewater Facial Toner

Step 6: Deep Condition Your Hair Naturally

Action:

Apply coconut oil to hair ends and leave for 30+ minutes before rinsing.

Tips & Hacks:

For extra shine, add rosemary oil (boosts hair growth, too!).

If hair is extra dry, sleep with the oil in (use a shower cap).

Favorite Oils:

Nutiva Organic Coconut Oil

Mielle Rosemary Mint Oil

Step 7: Track Progress & Plan Your Next Swaps

Action:

Keep a simple beauty journal to track skin and hair changes.

Tips & Hacks:

Set small goals—swap one product per week for a gradual detox.

Stay inspired—follow holistic beauty experts for natural skincare tips.

Favorite Tools:

Notion Template for Skin Tracking

Skin Bliss App

EXAMPLE 7 DAY PLAN

This 7-day beauty reset helps you transition to a cleaner, more natural skincare routine—without feeling overwhelmed. Each day focuses on one simple swap or habit, so by the end of the week, you'll have hydrated, nourished skin and a streamlined routine that works with your body, not against it.

How to Use This Plan:

Follow one step per day—easy, realistic changes add up!

No pressure to be perfect—just focus on progress.

Replace products gradually—no need to throw everything out at once.

Day 1	HYDRATE INSIDE AND OUT
	Glowing skin starts from within!
Action:	Drink ½ your body weight in ounces of water today.
	Apply coconut oil or shea butter post-shower to lock in hydration.
	Bonus: Add electrolytes (like **LMNT**) or a pinch of sea salt for better water absorption.
Impact:	Proper hydration = plumper, softer, and more radiant skin with fewer fine lines.

Day 2	DETOX YOUR SKINCARE PRODUCTS
	Out with the toxins, in with the clean beauty!
Action:	Scan your current beauty products using the Yuka App or Think Dirty App.
	Toss anything with parabens, phthalates, sulfates, synthetic fragrance, or a Yuka score below 75.

Start with just ONE swap—like switching to a clean moisturiz-
er or face wash.

Impact: Reducing chemical exposure leads to less irritation, fewer
breakouts, and better long-term skin health.

Day 3   TRY A DIY FACE MASK

Nature's ingredients = powerful skincare!

Action: Make a simple honey + yogurt mask for hydration and gentle
exfoliation.

For extra benefits: Add turmeric (anti-inflammatory) or oats
(soothing).

Leave on for 15 minutes while you relax (or multitask!).

Impact: Skin feels refreshed, soft, and deeply nourished—without the
chemicals found in store-bought masks.

Day 4   SWAP YOUR CLEANSER FOR OIL CLEANSING

Ditch the harsh foaming cleansers—your skin will thank you!

Action: Switch to oil cleansing using jojoba oil, squalane oil,
or olive oil.

For acne-prone skin: Add a drop of tea tree oil.

For dry skin: Mix in a little argan oil.

Impact: Cleansing with oil removes makeup, hydrates the skin, and
balances natural oils—without stripping your face.

Day 5   ADD A HYDRATING MIST

A quick refresh = all-day glow!

Action: Spritz rosewater mist throughout the day to hydrate and
soothe your skin.

DIY version: Mix rosewater + aloe vera for an easy homemade mist.

Keep a small bottle in your bag for a quick skin refresh.

Impact:	Skin stays moisturized and balanced, even in dry weather or after a long day.

Day 6	**DEEP CONDITION YOUR HAIR NATURALLY**

Stronger, shinier hair—without silicones or sulfates!

Action:	Apply coconut oil or argan oil to the ends of your hair.

Leave on for at least 30 minutes (or overnight for deep conditioning).

For hair growth: Add rosemary oil to your scalp before washing.

Impact:	Nourishes dry, brittle hair and prevents split ends—without synthetic conditioners.

Day 7	**REFLECT & PLAN YOUR NEXT SWAPS**

Track progress & keep the glow going!

Action:	Check in: How does your skin/hair feel after a week of natural beauty swaps?

Write down what worked and what didn't.

Set one goal for next week—maybe switching to a clean deodorant or non-toxic makeup.

Impact:	Helps you stay consistent, track improvements, and make small but lasting beauty upgrades!

CLEAN BEAUTY = HEALTHY BEAUTY

Taking care of your skin and hair shouldn't feel like a science experiment.

By switching to simpler, more natural ingredients, you're not only protecting your health but also embracing your natural beauty in a way that feels good, not forced.

Start with one swap at a time, track what works, and enjoy the process of nourishing your skin naturally.

BONUS TIPS FOR AN ONGOING NATURAL BEAUTY ROUTINE

If You're Feeling Overwhelmed:

Swap one product at a time—no need to do it all at once.

Stick to 3-5 essential skincare products instead of a 12-step routine.

If You Struggle with Dry Skin:

Use a humidifier at night.

Sleep on a silk pillowcase to reduce friction and irritation.

If You Want to Detox Your Makeup Too:

Check **EWG's Skin Deep** Database for clean foundation & mascara swaps.

Try **RMS Beauty, Ilia, or Well People** for non-toxic makeup options. (Check out my recommended brands in the Appendix)

FAQ'S

Q: Do natural products really work?

Answer: Yes, and they're often gentler on your skin. Plus, many contain potent, plant-based ingredients.

Q: How long before I see results?

Answer: Most people notice softer, clearer skin within 2–4 weeks, depending on consistency.

Q: Can I replace everything at once?

Answer: No need to! Gradually swap out products as they run out to avoid overwhelming your skin and budget.

Q: What if I have sensitive skin?

Answer: Start with ultra-gentle options like aloe vera gel or oatmeal masks and patch-test everything first.

Q: Can I use natural products during pregnancy?

Answer: Yes, most natural products are safe, but always consult your healthcare provider first.

Q: Are DIY masks as effective as store-bought ones?

Answer: Absolutely, and they're often fresher and free from preservatives.

Q: Will my skin purge when switching to natural products?

Answer: Some mild breakouts might happen as your skin adjusts, but it's temporary.

Q: Is coconut oil good for all skin types?

Answer: Not always—those with acne-prone skin might find it too heavy. Try jojoba or grapeseed oil instead.

Q: How can I ensure my products are truly natural?

Answer: Look for certifications like USDA Organic or verified non-toxic labels.

Q: Can natural beauty care really save money?

Answer: Yes! Many DIY options cost pennies compared to store-bought products.

What Comes Next

Okay. You've made it to the end of the book—but this is not the end of the journey.

You've learned the *why*. You've got the *how*. Now, the only thing left? *Action*.

And I know—it's easy to get stuck in the 'thinking about it' phase. But trust me, waiting for the 'perfect time' to start is like waiting for your toddler to magically stop asking 'why?' every two minutes. *It's not happening.*

So here's my challenge to you: If you haven't already…pick one protocol. Just one. Start today. Not tomorrow, not next week. TODAY!

It doesn't have to be big. It doesn't have to be perfect. It just has to be *something for you*.

Because the reality is—your health, your energy, your ability to enjoy motherhood—*it's in your hands*. No doctor, no pill, no quick fix is going to do this for you. *You* are the answer. You're the powerhouse matriarch.

THE NEXT STEP IS SIMPLE
SCAN THE QR CODE TO JOIN
THE MOVEMENT

*Unlock real strategies to heal your body, calm
your mind, and reclaim your power.*

www.thereginasteele.com

Appendix

Welcome to the Mother F*cked Appendix

Think of this as your survival stash. When life hits the fan (or your toddler throws sweet potatoes at the wall), this section has your back. It's loaded with real food recipes that don't suck, no-BS nutrition advice that won't bore you to death, practical mom hacks for dining out without wrecking your gut, and resources that prove you're not crazy—you're just carrying the weight of a broken system. Bookmark this part, dog-ear the pages, spill coffee on it—whatever. Just use it. This is your go-to toolkit for doing motherhood your way, not the way they say you should.

APPENDIX TABLE OF CONTENTS

Because flipping through chaos should at least be organized.

Appendix A: Real Food Recipes That Don't Suck

- ▶ Coconut Breakfast Parfait
- ▶ Avocado Toast
- ▶ Overnight Oats
- ▶ Mediterranean Quinoa Salad

- ► Sausage & Potato Soup
- ► Turkey & Avocado Wrap
- ► Chicken & Veggie Stir Fry
- ► White Bean & Mushroom Stew
- ► The Bliss Bowl
- ► Fermented Carrots
- ► Spiced Nuts
- ► Carrot Cake Bites

Appendix B: Nutrition & Pantry Cheat Sheet

- ► Cold Pantry Essentials
- ► Dry Pantry Power Players
- ► Nutrition Breakdown (Proteins, Fats, Grains, Fiber)
- ► Meal Prep Tips & Hacks
- ► Dining Out Without Losing Your Sh*t

Appendix C: The Helpers

- ► Journal Prompts (For When You're Stuck or Losing It)
- ► Self-Care Ideas That Actually Fit into Mom Life
- ► Clean Product Brands for Skin, Beauty & Sanity

Appendix D: Real Talk Research

- ► Economic Impacts (aka receipts for how broken the system is)
- ► Stats That'll Make You Rethink Everything (Backed by Science)

Appendix A: Real Food Recipes That Don't Suck

BREAKFAST IDEAS

COCONUT BREAKFAST PARFAIT

Creamy. Dreamy. No dairy demons.
Makes: 4 (8 oz mason jars)

You'll Need:
- ► 2 cans (15 oz) full-fat organic coconut milk
- ► 2.5 tbsp maple syrup
- ► 1.5 tsp cinnamon
- ► ½ tsp vanilla extract (or vegan baker's vanilla)
- ► ½ cup chia seeds
- ► Pinch of salt

Optional Toppings:
- ► Homemade jam (see note below)
- ► Granola (store-bought or homemade gluten-free)
- ► Nuts (pecans or walnuts = chef's kiss)
- ► Fresh berries (strawberries + raspberries are elite)
- ► Chopped fruit (apples, pears, etc.)

How to Make It:

1. Whisk all ingredients together in a bowl until creamy. *(Or blend everything but chia seeds, then stir them in afterward)*

2. Pour into jars or keep in a big bowl.

3. Refrigerate overnight. By morning, it's pudding perfection.

4. Top with whatever you're vibing with, or eat it as-is.

   Note: Homemade Jam Hack
   Add 1 chopped pear, 2 cups berries, 3 tbsp honey (or maple/coconut sugar), and 1 tbsp lemon juice to a pot. Simmer until juicy, blend it up, and store for up to 2 weeks in the fridge.

AVOCADO TOAST THAT DOESN'T SUCK

Because basic can still be badass.
Makes: 4 servings (2 tbsp each)

You'll Need:

- ► 1 medium avocado

- ► 1 tbsp chopped parsley

- ► 1 tbsp chopped green onions

- ► 3 tsp fresh lemon juice (yes, FRESH—not the bottle nonsense)

- ► 1 tsp olive oil

- ► Salt + pepper to taste

Topping Ideas:

Radishes, peppers, kalamata olives, nuts, seeds—whatever makes your gut (and taste buds) happy.

How to Make It:
1. Toss everything into a bowl.
2. Mash + mix. That's it.
3. Spread on toast, top with flair, and you're out the door.

OVERNIGHT OATS
(AKA THE LAZY BREAKFAST HERO)

Make once, eat all week. Mom win.
Prep Time: 5 minutes Lasts: Up to 5 days in the fridge

You'll Need (Per Jar):
▶ ½ cup gluten-free old-fashioned oats
▶ ⅛ tsp cinnamon
▶ 1 tsp honey (or maple syrup if you're watching that blood sugar)
▶ 2 tsp raisins
▶ Almond milk (or whatever non-dairy milk you're into)

How to Make It:
1. Line up 5 jars like a kitchen boss.
2. Using a funnel (optional but helps), add oats, cinnamon, honey, and raisins.
3. Pour milk to the top—don't freak if you need to top it off later.
4. Screw on lids, shake, and refrigerate.
5. In the AM: stir, top with nuts/seeds/fruit/whatever is easy, and go.

LUNCH IDEAS —quick, nourishing, and mom-tested (aka you can eat it standing up, hiding in the pantry, or in your car)

MEDITERRANEAN QUINOA SALAD

Basically a vacation in a bowl—but cheaper, faster, and with fewer crying children.

You'll Need:
- ► 1 cup baby kale (torn)
- ► 1 cup cooked quinoa (cooled)
- ► ½ cucumber, diced
- ► 2 tsp chopped kalamata olives (or more—always more)
- ► 1 green onion, diced (yes, use the white and green parts)
- ► 1 tsp chopped fresh parsley (don't you dare use dried)

Dressing:
- ► 1 tbsp olive oil
- ► 1 tbsp fresh lemon juice (I usually do more, because flavor)
- ► Salt + pepper to taste

Optional Toppings:
- ► Feta cheese
- ► Chopped chicken
- ► Peppers, beets, artichokes, crunchy chickpeas

How to Make It:
1. Toss the kale, quinoa, cucumber, olives, onion, and parsley in a big bowl.

2. Whisk the dressing ingredients in a separate bowl.

3. Pour dressing over the salad and toss again.

4. Top with whatever you've got on hand and devour.

SAUSAGE & POTATO SOUP

Comfort food that doesn't make you feel like a bloated marshmallow.
Serves: 6–8

You'll Need:
► 5 cups turkey or chicken broth (turkey is the crowd favorite)

► ¼ cup chopped parsley

► 1 sprig rosemary

► 1 bay leaf

► 1 lb ground pork or pork sausage (we use MOINK, seasoned with sage + pepper)

► 1 medium white onion, diced

► 1 large carrot, sliced

► 2 garlic cloves, minced

► 3 cups diced potatoes (red is great, but any kind works)

► ¼ tsp pepper

► 2 tbsp olive oil

► Salt to taste

How to Make It:
► Heat olive oil in a soup pot.

► Add sausage, onions, and carrots. Sauté until onions are soft.

► Add garlic + potatoes and stir for 1 minute.

► Pour in broth, herbs, and seasonings. Bring to a boil, then simmer until potatoes are tender.

► Add salt and pepper to taste, serve warm, and brace for happy bellies.

TURKEY & AVOCADO WRAP

For when you have zero time and one hand.

You'll Need:

► 1 whole-grain tortilla

► 3 slices turkey breast

► ½ avocado, sliced

► Handful of spinach

► 1 tbsp Greek yogurt

► 1 tsp mustard

► Salt + pepper

How to Make It:

1. Spread Greek yogurt + mustard on the tortilla.

2. Layer turkey, avocado, and spinach.

3. Season, roll, slice in half, and boom—done.

DINNER IDEAS —healthy, hearty, and actually enjoyable (even if you're microwaving it while yelling "GET IN THE SHOWER" down the hallway)

CHICKEN & VEGGIE STIR FRY

Because some nights, you just need to throw everything in a pan and call it good.

You'll Need:

- ► 2 chicken breasts, diced
- ► 2 tbsp olive oil
- ► 1 cup broccoli florets
- ► 1 red bell pepper, sliced
- ► 1 carrot, sliced
- ► ½ cup snap peas
- ► 2 tbsp soy sauce (or tamari for gluten-free moms)
- ► 1 tsp garlic powder
- ► 1 tsp ginger powder
- ► 2 cups cooked brown rice

How to Make It:

1. Heat oil in a large pan.
2. Add chicken and cook until browned and no longer pink (5–7 min).
3. Toss in all the veggies and stir-fry for another 5–6 minutes until tender-crisp.
4. Stir in soy sauce, garlic, and ginger. Cook for another 2 minutes.
5. Serve over rice. Boom. Dinner's done and everyone's fed.

WHITE BEAN & MUSHROOM STEW

It's cozy. It's rich. And nobody misses the meat.

You'll Need:

- ► 3 tbsp vegan butter or olive oil

- ► 1 medium onion, diced
- ► 1 lb mushrooms (shiitake + cremini are the dream team), sliced
- ► ¾ tsp dried thyme
- ► ¾ tsp dried rosemary
- ► ¾ tsp sea salt + pepper
- ► 4 garlic cloves, minced
- ► 2 tbsp cornstarch or flour
- ► 2 tsp tamari or soy sauce
- ► 1 tbsp Dijon mustard
- ► 3 cups veggie broth
- ► 1 lb baby potatoes, cubed
- ► 2 cans white beans, drained + rinsed
- ► 2 cups unsweetened non-dairy milk (almond works great)

How to Make It:

1. In a big pot, sauté onions in butter/oil until soft.
2. Add mushrooms + herbs. Cook 7–10 min until they brown and lose moisture.
3. Add garlic. Stir for 1 min.
4. Sprinkle in cornstarch, stir to coat. Add tamari + Dijon.
5. Pour in broth + potatoes. Simmer until potatoes are tender (15–20 min).
6. Add beans + milk. Simmer another 10–15 min until thickened.
7. Taste, adjust seasoning, serve warm. Refrigerates or freezes like a dream.

THE BLISS BOWL

A nourishing bowl that feels like a hug and tastes like heaven.

Base:
- ► 1 cup cooked quinoa or brown rice

Protein:
- ► ½ cup roasted chickpeas (seasoned with paprika + garlic)
- ► 1 soft-boiled egg (optional but bossy)

Veggies:
- ► 1 cup steamed broccoli
- ► ½ cup roasted sweet potatoes
- ► Handful of spinach or arugula

Toppings:
- ► ¼ avocado, sliced
- ► 1 tbsp sunflower or pumpkin seeds
- ► Sprinkle of pomegranate seeds

Dressing:
- ► 2 tbsp tahini
- ► 1 tbsp lemon juice
- ► 1 tsp maple syrup
- ► 1–2 tbsp water (to thin)
- ► Pinch of sea salt + pepper

How to Make It:
1. Start with your grain base.
2. Pile on the protein + veggies.
3. Add toppings like you mean it.
4. Whisk dressing ingredients and drizzle that creamy goodness all over.
5. Shovel it in with pride.

SNACK IDEAS

FERMENTED CARROTS (THE GUT-GLOWING CRUNCH)
Your microbiome's new BFF—and oddly addictive.

You'll Need:
- ▶ 3–4 large carrots (peeled + sliced into sticks)
- ▶ 1 cup water (filtered!)
- ▶ 1 tbsp sea salt (no iodine, no regrets)
- ▶ 1–2 garlic cloves, smashed
- ▶ Optional add-ins: peppercorns, dill, red pepper flakes for heat

How to Make It:
1. Dissolve salt in the water to make a simple brine.
2. Pack carrots, garlic, and extras into a wide-mouth mason jar.
3. Pour brine over everything until fully submerged.
4. Cover with a lid or cloth + rubber band.
5. Let sit at room temp for 3–5 days (burp the jar daily to avoid explosions).
6. Once tangy + bubbly, pop it in the fridge and snack away.

SPICED NUTS
Aka: "The reason you're still functioning at 4 p.m."

You'll Need:
- ▶ 3 cups mixed nuts (raw + unsalted)
- ▶ 2 tbsp avocado oil (or coconut oil)

- ► 1 tbsp maple syrup
- ► 2 tsp smoked paprika
- ► 1 tsp ground cinnamon
- ► 1 tsp chili powder
- ► ½ tsp salt
- ► Dash of cayenne if you like it wild

How to Make It:
1. Preheat oven to 300°F.
2. Mix everything in a big bowl until nuts are fully coated.
3. Spread on a parchment-lined baking sheet.
4. Roast for 20–25 min, stirring halfway through.
5. Cool completely before storing in a jar (and hiding from your kids).

CARROT CAKE BITES
They taste like dessert but work like fuel. Mom trickery at its finest.

You'll Need:
- ► 1 cup shredded carrots
- ► ¾ cup dates (softened in hot water for 5 min)
- ► 1 cup unsweetened shredded coconut
- ► ¾ cup walnuts or cashews
- ► ½ tsp cinnamon
- ► ¼ tsp nutmeg
- ► Pinch of salt
- ► 1 tsp vanilla extract
- ► 1–2 tbsp almond or oat flour (if needed for consistency)

How to Make It:

1. Pulse everything in a food processor until it clumps.

2. Roll into bite-sized balls.

3. Store in the fridge up to 7 days (if they last that long).

4. Optional: roll in extra coconut flakes to look extra fancy.

For more recipes and ideas check out my website at **www.thereginasteele.com**

Appendix B: Nutrition & Pantry Cheat Sheet

aka your "how to not burn out and still eat like a damn queen" manual

PANTRY CHEAT SHEET

COLD PANTRY MVPS (FRIDGE ESSENTIALS)

Because when your fridge is stocked with the right stuff, survival is more likely.

Fermented Foods: sauerkraut, pickles (no vinegar ones), kimchi, coconut yogurt, kefir

Produce: berries, greens, carrots, celery, lemons, cucumbers

Oils & Spreads: coconut oil, almond butter, tahini, grass-fed butter/ghee

Protein: nitrate-free bacon, wild-caught salmon, organic eggs, bone broth

Condiments: coconut aminos, mustard, dairy-free pesto, cashew cream

Prep Must-Haves: cooked grains, roasted veggies, pre-washed greens, chopped herbs

DRY PANTRY POWER PLAYERS (SHELF-STABLE LIFESAVERS)

Because let's be honest—some nights dinner is a can + a prayer.

- ► Gluten-free oats
- ► Brown rice + quinoa
- ► Canned beans (rinse 'em)
- ► Raw nuts + seeds
- ► Dried herbs/spices
- ► Avocado oil + olive oil
- ► Coconut milk (full-fat, always)
- ► Almond flour + coconut flour
- ► Apple cider vinegar + raw honey
- ► Sea salt, black pepper, garlic powder, turmeric, cinnamon

Snack Smarts
For when the hangry hits but the drive-thru isn't an option.

- ► Organic popcorn
- ► Freeze-dried fruit
- ► Paleo bars (check the damn ingredients)
- ► Trail mix (DIY if possible)
- ► Chia packs
- ► Rice cakes + almond butter
- ► Seaweed snacks

Beverage Basics
Hydration = Energy. Dehydration = You snapping at your kids for breathing too loud.

- ► Herbal teas (peppermint, ginger, chamomile)
- ► LMNT or other clean electrolytes
- ► Coconut water (no added sugar)
- ► Filtered water with lemon, cucumber, or mint
- ► Bone broth (counts as sipping gold)

NUTRITION BREAKDOWN: WHAT YOUR BODY ACTUALLY WANTS

Protein: The Building Block You Keep Forgetting About
(And no, coffee isn't a protein.)

Your energy, mood, metabolism, muscle repair, hormones, and even your hair depend on it.

Top Protein Picks (Mix & Match):
- ► Organic chicken or turkey
- ► Wild-caught salmon, sardines, mackerel
- ► Grass-fed beef
- ► Eggs (yes, the yolks too)
- ► Bone broth
- ► Hemp seeds, chia seeds
- ► Lentils, chickpeas, black beans
- ► Tempeh, organic tofu
- ► Protein powders (check for crap ingredients—aim clean, no fillers or sweeteners)

Mom Hack: Add protein to every meal and snack. No exceptions. Tired? Start here.

HEALTHY FATS: THE STUFF THAT FEEDS YOUR BRAIN (AND KEEPS YOU FULL)
This is not the '90s. Fat doesn't make you fat—stress, sugar, and starvation do.

Best Fats for Fuel:
- ► Avocados
- ► Nuts (walnuts, almonds, cashews)

- Seeds (pumpkin, flax, chia, sunflower)
- Extra virgin olive oil
- Coconut oil or butter
- Ghee
- Fatty fish (hello, omega-3s)

Mom Hack: Add 1–2 healthy fats to each meal—your hormones and brain will thank you.

GRAINS + CARBS: YES, YOU'RE ALLOWED TO EAT THEM

Just pick ones that don't wreck your blood sugar and mood.

Smart Carbs:
- Brown rice, wild rice
- Quinoa
- Steel-cut or gluten-free rolled oats
- Sweet potatoes, squash
- Buckwheat
- Amaranth
- Chickpea or lentil pasta

Mom Hack: Pair carbs with protein or fat to avoid crashing by 2pm (or rage-texting your spouse).

FIBER: YOUR GUT'S LOVE LANGUAGE

Most moms are more fiber-deprived than sleep-deprived (which is saying a lot).

High-Fiber Heroes:
- Leafy greens (spinach, kale, arugula)
- Berries (raspberries, blackberries, blueberries)

- ► Chia seedsFlaxseeds
- ► Lentils + beans
- ► Broccoli, cauliflower, Brussels sprouts
- ► Apples, pears (with skin)

Mom Hack: If you're not pooping daily, you're not detoxing. Up your fiber. Hydrate. Move.

MEAL PREP & DINING OUT: MOM SURVIVAL STRATEGIES

Real Talk: Meal Prep Isn't Just for Gym Bros and Pinterest Influencers

It's your *bare minimum strategy* for eating like an adult even when your life is chaos.

Basic Mom-Approved Meal Prep Strategy:

1. Pick 2 Proteins – Bake a tray of chicken thighs and toss a pot roast in the slow cooker. Done.

2. Prep 2 Grains – Think quinoa + brown rice. Make extra and freeze some.

3. Chop All the Veggies – Do it once, not 6 different nights while your toddler is licking the fridge.

4. Make One Dressing or Sauce – Tahini-lemon. Balsamic-olive oil. Whatever makes things taste better fast.

5. Hard-Boil Eggs – The original grab-and-go snack.

6. ortion Out Some Snack Bags – DIY trail mix, sliced veggies, spiced nuts.

Mom Hack: Batch roast EVERYTHING on one night while

you binge your latest show. It's called multitasking and it's a damn art form.

DINING OUT WITHOUT DESTROYING YOUR GUT OR GUILT

You're allowed to eat out and still care about your health. Here's how to do both.

RESTAURANT SURVIVAL TIPS:

❒ **Scan the menu beforehand**
Saves time and decisions when you're hangry and overstimulated.

❒ **Skip the bread basket**
Unless it's artisanal sourdough and worth the bloat.

❒ **Protein first**
Look for grilled, roasted, or baked options.

❒ **Build a bowl or plate**
hink protein + veggies + healthy fat.

❒ **Ask for modifications**
You're paying, not begging. Sub the fries. Ditch the sauce. Own it.

❒ **Watch the sauces + dressings**
Ask for them on the side (and yes, it's okay to be *that* person).

❒ **Hydrate before + after**
Dining out dehydrates you more than your toddler's tantrum.

DRINKS

☐ Go for sparkling water with citrus, kombucha, herbal iced teas, or one clean cocktail (and avoid sugary mixers).

☐ If you're drinking wine: hydrate between sips and take your magnesium before bed.

Appendix C: The Helpers

Because you can't pour from an empty cup…
and yours has a damn crack in it.

JOURNAL PROMPTS (FOR WHEN YOU'RE STUCK, SPINNING, OR JUST NEED A MOMENT)

Think of this as the mental cleanse your brain's been begging for. What is something I actually need right now?

1. What is draining me that I have the power to pause, limit, or say no to?

2. What would I do with one uninterrupted hour just for me?

3. What does "healthy" feel like in my body—not just look like?

4. What am I proud of surviving—even if no one noticed?

5. What part of motherhood do I want to redefine on my terms?

6. What lies about womanhood, success, or health am I ready to stop believing?

7. What would it feel like to give myself more grace than guilt?

Mom Hack: Journal like no one's reading. Because no one is (unless you leave it out and your toddler uses it as a coloring book).

SELF-CARE ROUTINES THAT ACTUALLY WORK FOR MOMS

Not the "3-hour Sunday reset" nonsense. Real, doable rituals that refill your tank

DAILY MICRO-MOMENTS:

▶ Morning: Open a window + breathe deep for 1 minute (yes, just that).

▶ Midday: Step outside + stretch your arms to the sky. Bonus if you don't scream

▶ Evening: Put on magnesium lotion, listen to music, and ignore your phone.

WEEKLY SUPPORT:

▶ Take a solo walk—no kids, no stroller, no guilt.

▶ Make one nourishing meal just for you—not leftovers, not kid scraps.

▶ Do something creative (even if it's reorganizing your junk drawer to music).

▶ Set a boundary and stick to it. (Say no. Then don't explain.)

CLEAN PRODUCT BRAND FAVORITES

Because you deserve skincare that doesn't mess with your hormones.

CLEAN PRODUCT BRAND FAVORITES

SKIN & MAKEUP:

- ► **Beautycounter:** Non-toxic, high-performing skincare & makeup

- ► **Ilia:** Clean makeup with skin-loving ingredients

- ► **Cocokind:** Budget-friendly + effective skincare

- ► **Primally Pure:** Natural deodorant that actually works

- ► **Alitura:** Luxurious AF and totally non-toxic

BODY & HAIR:

- ► **Innersense:** Salon-worthy haircare with clean ingredients

- ► **OSEA:** Ocean-based, spa-like skincare line

- ► **Earth Mama Organics:** Especially great for postpartum + sensitive skin

- ► **Native:** Cucumber Mint is clean and smells like a vacation in a bottle

Mom Hack: You don't have to swap it all at once. Replace one product at a time when it runs out— no stress.

Appendix D: Real Talk Resources

*Stats + Studies That Prove Moms
Are Systemically Screwed*

Welcome to your "see, it's not just me" section. When you need backup for why you're tired, burnt out, or rage-crying on a Tuesday, this is it.

BURNOUT IS REAL, AND MOMS ARE GROUND ZERO

▸ 88% of American moms say they feel more stressed now than before having kids. *(Source: Motherly State of Motherhood Survey)*

▸ 1 in 3 moms report feeling completely burned out, not just tired. *(American Psychological Association)*

▸ Maternal mental health issues (like anxiety + depression) have risen 300% in the last two decades.

Why It Matters: You're not just tired. You're carrying emotional labor, invisible tasks, and generational expectations—on zero sleep.

The Workload Math Is Wild

▸ Moms working full-time jobs still spend an additional 3.2 hours/day on household and child care responsibilities.

- ► That adds up to 98 extra hours/month—aka two and a half full-time jobs.

- ► And only 6% of working moms say they receive "most of the support" they need from their partner or employer. *(Pew Research Center, 2022)*

The Nervous System Wasn't Built For This Sh*t

Chronic stress—especially unmanaged "low-level" stress like multitasking, overstimulation, and emotional labor—leads to:

- ► Increased cortisol (which wrecks sleep, skin, energy, and hormones)

- ► Gut dysbiosis (a fancy way of saying your microbiome is under attack)

- ► Hormonal imbalance (hello, rage, exhaustion, and PMS from hell

- ► Suppressed immune function (aka, why you're always catching your kid's crud)

The Fix? Not another prescription. Not a 3-day juice cleanse. Not toxic positivity. It's nervous system regulation, support, boundaries, and real food.

And Let's Not Forget the Cost of "Trying to Be Okay"

- ► Women spend 10–15% more annually on healthcare than men—mostly on hormonal, autoimmune, and chronic conditions.

- ► The U.S. spends more on healthcare per person than any other developed nation—but ranks dead last for maternal outcomes. *(Source: Commonwealth Fund)*

So yeah, it's not just you. You've been motherf*cked by a system that expects you to run a home, raise humans, maintain a career, and smile through it all. This book? It's your rebuttal.

Exercises Connection To Postpartum Recovery

Oh, absolutely—and not just because you're chasing after your toddler or doing 50 squats every time you bend down to pick up a pacifier. Postpartum exercise can be a game-changer for new moms, helping you rebuild strength, boost your mood, and feel more like a functional human again. Here is how:

Physical Strengthening

Pregnancy and childbirth do a number on your body—hello, ab separation and back pain! Postpartum exercise helps rebuild those major muscle groups, especially your core and back. Think of it as fortifying the fortress that is you, so you can survive endless baby-holding marathons and stroller-hauling heroics.

Mood Enhancement

If you've ever felt like crying into your coffee after a sleepless night, exercise might just be your new best friend. Moving your body releases endorphins—the "feel-good" hormones—that can help combat postpartum depression and anxiety. It's basically free therapy, minus the couch and awkward small talk.

Increased Energy Levels

Yes, I know it sounds counterintuitive when you're already running on fumes, but regular exercise can actually boost your energy. A quick walk or some light strength training can do wonders to shake off the zombie mom vibes and help you feel like you can take on the day (or at least the next diaper blowout).

Faster Recovery Time

Want to feel like yourself again a little sooner? Safe, gradual exercise helps rebuild strength and stamina, making daily tasks—like carrying a car seat that weighs as much as a small pony—a little easier. Just take it slow and listen to your body. No medals for overdoing it!

Social Interaction

Group exercise classes or mommy-and-me workouts aren't just good for your body—they're great for your sanity. Connecting with other moms who get it can make a world of difference, whether you're bonding over burpees or laughing about how your baby spit up on your yoga mat.

EXERCISES IMPACT ON SLEEP

If there's one thing every mom wants more of, it's sleep. And while I can't promise exercise will magically make your baby sleep through the night (sorry), it can help you sleep better when you finally get the chance. Here's how:

Hormonal Benefits

Exercise boosts melatonin, your body's natural sleep hormone, helping you fall asleep faster and stay asleep longer. Think of it as nature's gentle nudge toward dreamland.

Stress Reduction

You know that wired-but-exhausted feeling that keeps you staring at the ceiling at 3 AM? Exercise can help with that. By reducing stress hormones like cortisol, it creates a calmer mental state that's perfect for drifting off (when the baby finally gives you a break).

Physical Benefits for Better Sleep

Strength training and cardio don't just tone your body—they can also improve your sleep quality while easing postpartum anxiety or depression. A few push-ups or a brisk walk can work wonders for both your muscles and your mood.

Better Sleep Patterns

Exercise helps regulate your internal clock, making it easier to establish a healthy sleep-wake cycle. It's like a natural reset button for those unpredictable postpartum schedules.

Overall Sleep Quality

The relationship between sleep and exercise is a two-way street. Better sleep makes it easier to exercise, and regular exercise improves your sleep. That's a win-win!

SLEEP 411

Prioritizing sleep is one way to flip that script and take care of yourself—because when mom's thriving, everyone benefits. Check these out:

1. **Postpartum Sleep and Depression:** Studies show that sleep deprivation significantly increases the risk of postpartum depression (PPD) in **10 to 20% new moms.** Although many in the integrative space know this to be higher.

2. **Hormones and Sleep:** Research highlights the impact of hormonal changes on sleep quality, especially during pregnancy and postpartum. Impacting appetite and weight.

3. **Cognitive Benefits:** Sleep is essential for decision-making and multitasking—two skills every mom needs in the chaos of daily life.

4. **Physical Health:** Sleep helps regulate weight, immune function, and heart health, all critical for busy moms.

5. **Immune Function:** Sleep enhances the production of cytokines and the function of T cells, which are **critical for the body's defense** against infections.

6. **Family Sleep Patterns:** Research shows a strong link between parent and child sleep habits, emphasizing the importance of leading by example. Plus, moms are able to engage positively to create a supportive environment…aka: mom's not snappy!

And as you probably already know: these sleep struggles don't magically disappear after the newborn phase. Research shows new parents can face up to six years of disrupted sleep, with the rock-bottom phase hitting hard around the three-month mark. The good news? Knowing the reality is the first step in figuring out how to survive, and maybe even thrive, on less sleep.

Citation List

Harris Poll, https://www.cvshealth.com/news/mental-health/the-mental-health-crisis-of-working-moms.html#:~:text=And%20mothers%20who%20remained%20at,even%20working%20fathers%20(35%25).

Forbes, https://www.forbes.com/councils/forbesbusinesscouncil/2024/05/22/why-is-there-still-a-gender-wage-gap/.

riskology.co, https://www.riskology.co/importance-of-community/.

The American Journal of Clinical Nutrition, https://ajcn.nutrition.org/action/consumeSharedSessionAction?JSESSIONID=aaa7OpQAKX02F-cbuPyPfz&MAID=IzCN8lyy5wM5r%2FdcNc7mmw%3D%3D&ORIGIN=210246975&RD=RD&exp=O%252FqnWKdv%252FTtGSI2Zrsvi-JQ%253D%253D.

Breastcancer.org - Breast Cancer Information and Support, http://breastcancer.org. Accessed 27 February 2025.

https://qalo.com/blogs/qalo-life/12-at-home-workouts-to-do-with-your-kids.

The Vision Council: Register Now for the Lab Leadership Forum, https://thevisioncouncil.org/. Accessed 27 February 2025.

The Association Between Social Isolation and Health: An Analysis of Parent–Adolescent Dyads from the Family Life, Activity, Sun, Health, and Eating Study, 28 October 2019, https://www.ncbi.nlm.nih.gov/pmc/articles/PMC7222048/. Accessed 27 February 2025.

A systematic review of parental burnout and related factors among parents, 5 February 2024, https://www.ncbi.nlm.nih.gov/pmc/articles/PMC10840230/. Accessed 27 February 2025.

Alharbi, Mutasim D., et al. "The relationship between fatigue, sleep quality, resilience, and the risk of postpartum depression: an emphasis on maternal mental health - BMC Psychology." BMC Psychology, 13 January 2023, https://bmcpsychology.biomedcentral.com/articles/10.1186/s40359-023-01043-3. Accessed 27 February 2025.

Alimujiang, Aliya, et al. "Association Between Life Purpose and Mortality Among US Adults Older Than 50 Years." JAMA, JAMA, 2019, https://jamanetwork.com/journals/jamanetworkopen/fullarticle/2734064?utm_source=For_The_Media&utm_medium=referral&utm_campaign=ftm_links&utm_term=052419.

"Americans' Views of Health Care Costs, Access, and Quality." PubMed Central, https://www.ncbi.nlm.nih.gov/pmc/articles/PMC2690297/. Accessed 27 February 2025.

Amici, Federica, et al. "Maternal stress, child behavior and the promotive role of older siblings." BMC, 2022, https://bmcpublichealth.biomedcentral.com/articles/10.1186/s12889-022-13261-2#:~:text=Maternal%20stress%2C%20child%20behavior,promotive%20role%20of%20older.

Anderson, Gerard, and Jane Horvath. "The Growing Burden of Chronic Disease in America." NIH, vol. 119, 2004, https://www.ncbi.nlm.nih.gov/pmc/articles/PMC1497638/pdf/15158105.pdf#:~:text=The%20number%20of%20people%20with,to%20people%20with%20chronic%20conditions.

Archer, Edward, et al. "Maternal Inactivity: 45-Year Trends in Mothers' Use of Time." Mayo Clinic, 2013, https://www.mayoclinicproceedings.org/article/S0025-6196(13)00828-8/fulltext.

"The association between sedentary behaviour and risk of anxiety: a systematic review - BMC Public Health." BMC Public Health, 19 June 2015, https://bmcpublichealth.biomedcentral.com/articles/10.1186/s12889-015-1843-x. Accessed 27 February 2025.

Auman-Bauer, Kristie. "Parental stress and child behavior health impacts." Penn State, 2016, https://www.psu.edu/news/research/story/parental-stress-and-child-behavior-health-impacts#:~:text=%E2%80%9CMaternal%20stress%20has%20been,on%20the%20well%2Dbeing%20of.

Berthelon, Matias, et al. "Maternal stress during pregnancy and early childhood development." ScienceDirect, 2021, https://www.sciencedirect.com/science/article/abs/pii/S1570677X2100071X#:~:text=2021%20%2D%20In%20utero,that%20the%20effects%20are.

"Bones." Better Health Channel, https://www.betterhealth.vic.gov.au/health/conditionsandtreatments/bones. Accessed 27 February 2025.

Brody, Debra J., and Qiuping Gu. "Products - Data Briefs - Number 377 - September 2020." CDC, 4 September 2020, https://www.cdc.gov/nchs/products/databriefs/db377.htm. Accessed 27 February 2025.

Buechler, Jessica. "The Loneliness Epidemic Persists: A Post-Pandemic Look at the State of Loneliness among U.S. Adults." The Cigna Group Newsroom, 26 May 2022, https://newsroom.thecignagroup.com/loneliness-epidemic-persists-post-pandemic-look. Accessed 27 February 2025.

"Calcium and Bone Health." HelpGuide.org, 30 September 2024, https://www.helpguide.org/wellness/nutrition/calcium-and-bone-health. Accessed 27 February 2025.

"Cancer explained." Better Health Channel, https://www.betterhealth.vic.gov.au/health/conditionsandtreatments/cancer. Accessed 27 February 2025.

Carnahan, Jill. "Functional Medicine Restores Healthy Function by Treating the Root Causes of Disease." | The Institute for Functional Medicine, https://www.ifm.org/functional-medicine/what-is-functional-medicine/. Accessed 27 February 2025.

Cashin, Ali. "Loneliness in America: How the Pandemic Has Deepened an Epidemic of Loneliness and What We Can Do About It." Making Caring Common, 9 February 2021, https://mcc.gse.harvard.edu/reports/loneliness-in-america. Accessed 27 February 2025.

Chen, I-Chun. "Americans, Mostly Women, Spent 12 Billion on Plastic Surgery Last Year." NAMD, 2023, https://www.namd.org/journal-chronicle-of-medicine/1878-americans-mostly-women-spent-12-billion-on-plastic-surgery-last-year.html.

"Choosing Healthy Fats." HelpGuide.org, 16 January 2025, https://www.helpguide.org/wellness/nutrition/choosing-healthy-fats. Accessed 27 February 2025.

"Choosing Healthy Fats." HelpGuide.org, 16 January 2025, https://www.helpguide.org/wellness/nutrition/choosing-healthy-fats. Accessed 27 February 2025.

"Choosing Healthy Protein." HelpGuide.org, 7 June 2024, https://www.helpguide.org/wellness/nutrition/choosing-healthy-protein. Accessed 27 February 2025.

Cimon-Paquet, Catherine, et al. "Early parent–child relationships and child sleep at school age." ScienceDirect, 2019, https://www.sciencedirect.com/science/article/abs/pii/S0193397318302521#:~:text=Parent%E2%80%93child%20relationships%20and%20child%20sleep.

The Cleveland Clinic. "5 Healthy Habits That Prevent Chronic Disease." The Cleveland Clinic, 2020.

Colditz, G. A. "Economic costs of obesity and inactivity." 1999, https://pubmed.ncbi.nlm.nih.gov/10593542/ "A comparison of fatigue and energy levels at 6 weeks and 14 to 19 months postpartum." PubMed, https://pubmed.ncbi.nlm.nih.gov/10887866/. Accessed 27 February 2025.

"Conventional Medicine Vs. Functional Medicine." Dr. Will Cole, https://drwillcole.com/functional-medicine-vs-conventional-medicine. Accessed 27 February 2025.

"Correlates of leisure-time physical activity during transitions to motherhood." National Library of Medicine, NIH, 2009, https://pubmed.ncbi.nlm.nih.gov/19485235/.

Crnic, Keith, et al. "Effects of Stress and Social Support on Mothers and Premature and Full-Term Infants." Jstor, vol. 54, no. 1, 1983, pp. 209-217, https://www.jstor.org/stable/1129878.

Damon, William, et al. "The Development of Purpose During Adolescence." Taylor & Francis, 2010, https://www.tandfonline.com/doi/abs/10.1207/S1532480XADS0703_2.

de Brito, Junio, et al. "Changes in Physical Activity and Sedentary Behaviors During COVID-19: Associations with Psychological Distress Among Mothers." NIH, 2021, https://www.ncbi.nlm.nih.gov/pmc/articles/PMC8605880/#:~:text=After%20controlling%20for%20sociodemographic%20factors,but%20not%20lower)%20levels%20of.

"Deep vein thrombosis." Better Health Channel, https://www.betterhealth.vic.gov.au/health/conditionsandtreatments/deep-vein-thrombosis. Accessed 27 February 2025.

De La Merced, Abby. "Ultra-Processed Foods And Mental Health." 2024, https://remedypsychiatry.com/ultra-processed-foods-and-mental-health/.

"Depression and anxiety: Exercise eases symptoms." Mayo Clinic, https://www.mayoclinic.org/diseases-conditions/depression/in-depth/depression-and-exercise/art-20046495. Accessed 27 February 2025.

"Diabetes." Better Health Channel, https://www.betterhealth.vic.gov.au/health/conditionsandtreatments/diabetes. Accessed 27 February 2025.

"Dietary Supplements: Benefits and Safety Precautions." HelpGuide.org, 27 September 2024, https://www.helpguide.org/wellness/nutrition/dietary-supplements. Accessed 27 February 2025.

Documenting Hope. "Autism Growth Rate: Projected." Documenting Hope, 2025, https://epidemicanswers.org/about-the-epidemic/the-startling-statistics. Accessed 17 05 2025

"The economic impact of untreated maternal mental health conditions in Texas - BMC Pregnancy and Childbirth." BMC Pregnancy and Childbirth, 12 September 2022, https://bmcpregnancychildbirth.biomedcentral.com/articles/10.1186/s12884-022-05001-6. Accessed 27 February 2025.

"The Effects of Prenatal Stress on Child Behavioural and Cognitive Outcomes Start at the Beginning." Encyclopedia on Early Childhood Development, 1 April 2019, https://www.child-encyclopedia.com/stress-and-pregnancy-prenatal-and-perinatal/according-experts/effects-prenatal-stress-child. Accessed 27 February 2025.

"The Effects of Prenatal Stress on Child Behavioural and Cognitive Outcomes Start at the Beginning." Encyclopedia on Early Childhood Development, 1 April 2019, https://www.child-encyclopedia.com/stress-and-pregnancy-prenatal-and-perinatal/according-experts/effects-prenatal-stress-child. Accessed 27 February 2025.

"Endocrine-disrupting chemicals and skin manifestations." PubMed, https://pubmed.ncbi.nlm.nih.gov/27363826/. Accessed 27 February 2025.

Epperson, C. Neill, et al. "Healthcare resource utilization and costs associated with postpartum depression among commercially insured households." Taylor & Francis, https://www.tandfonline.com/doi/full/10.1080/03007995.2020.1799772#:~:text=2020%20%2D%20The%20findings,extends%20beyond%20mothers.%20Moreover%2C.

Everett, Cara. "8 Best Weight Loss Programs Reviewed and Tested in 2024." 2024, https://www.helpguide.org/handbook/healthy-living/best-weight-loss-programs.

Ewens, Michael. "The $282 Billion Toll: Quantifying the Economic Impact of Mental Illness | Columbia Business School." Columbia Business School, 18 October 2024, https://business.columbia.edu/research-brief/economic-impact-mental-illness? Accessed 27 February 2025.

"Exercise During Pregnancy." ACOG, https://www.acog.org/womens-health/faqs/exercise-during-pregnancy. Accessed 27 February 2025.

"Exercising for Better Sleep." Johns Hopkins Medicine, https://www.hopkinsmedicine.org/health/wellness-and-prevention/exercising-for-better-sleep. Accessed 27 February 2025.

"FDA Drug Recall Statistics [Updated For 2024]." Lightfoot Law, PLLC, 1 April 2024, https://www.maylightfootlaw.com/blogs/fda-drug-recall-statistics/. Accessed 27 February 2025.

"5 Significant Drug Recalls in US History & Why They Happened." Handler, Henning & Rosenberg LLC, 14 March 2022, https://www.hhrlaw.com/blog/2019/october/5-significant-drug-recalls-in-us-history-why-the/. Accessed 27 February 2025.

Greenan, Shawn. "What is Functional Medicine? How Do I Find A Functional Medicine Practitioner?" Rupa Health, 2025, https://www.rupahealth.com/post/what-is-functional-medicine#:~:text=Functional%20medicine%20uses%20in%2Ddepth,focus%20on%20standard%20lab%20testing.

Harvard University. "The Nutrition Source: Sugary Drinks." Harvard School of Public Health, 2024.

"Health consequences of circadian disruption in humans and animal models." PubMed, https://pubmed.ncbi.nlm.nih.gov/23899601/. Accessed 27 February 2025.

Heiting, Gary. "How To Help Children Avoid Computer Vision Syndrome." All About Vision, https://www.allaboutvision.com/cvs/children-computer-vision-syndrome.htm. Accessed 27 February 2025.

"Help for Perinatal Individuals." Postpartum Support International, https://www.postpartum.net/get-help/help-for-moms/. Accessed 27 February 2025.

Hensley, Scott. "Annals Of The Obvious: Women Way More Tired Than Men." NPR, 12 April 2013, https://www.npr.org/sections/health-shots/2013/04/11/176936210/annals-of-the-obvious-women-way-more-tired-than-men. Accessed 27 February 2025.

Hill, Patrick, and Nicholas Turiano. "Purpose in Life as a Predictor of Mortality across Adulthood." 2014, https://www.ncbi.nlm.nih.gov/pmc/articles/PMC4224996/.

Holt-Lunstad, Julainne. "Loneliness and Social Isolation as Risk Factors for Mortality: A Meta-Analytic Review." Sage Journals, 2015, https://journals.sagepub.com/doi/10.1177/1745691614568352.

"How Sleep Deprivation Impacts Mental Health." Columbia University Department of Psychiatry, 16 March 2022, https://www.columbiapsychiatry.org/news/how-sleep-deprivation-affects-your-mental-health. Accessed 27 February 2025.

"How Sleep Deprivation Impacts Mental Health." Columbia University Department of Psychiatry, 16 March 2022, https://www.columbiapsychiatry.org/news/how-sleep-deprivation-affects-your-mental-health. Accessed 27 February 2025.

Huyett, Phillip, and Neil Bhattacharyya. "Incremental health care utilization and expenditures for sleep disorders in the United States." 2021, https://jcsm.aasm.org/doi/10.5664/jcsm.9392?

"Inactive mothers lead to inactive kids." New Zealand Herald, New Zealand Herald, 2014, https://www.nzherald.co.nz/lifestyle/inactive-mothers-lead-to-inactive-kids-study/YQXHTRLICZU5ZXDYFPAWWEVI4U/#google_vignette.

Isler, Amy. "Study: Maternal Stress Linked To Negative Health Outcomes for Kids." VeryWellHealth, 2021, https://www.verywellhealth.com/maternal-stress-linked-to-disease-development-in-children-5095761#:~:text=This%20response%20then%20triggers,children.%20Negative%20Health%20Effects.

Juby, Bethany. "Mental health: Definition, common disorders, early signs, and more." MedicalNewsToday, 22 March 2024, https://www.medicalnewstoday.com/articles/154543.php. Accessed 27 February 2025.

"'Just snap out of it' – the experience of loneliness in women with perinatal depression: a Meta-synthesis of qualitative studies - BMC Psychiatry." BMC Psychiatry, 28 February 2023, https://bmcpsychiatry.biomedcentral.com/articles/10.1186/s12888-023-04532-2. Accessed 27 February 2025.

"'Just snap out of it' – the experience of loneliness in women with perinatal depression: a Meta-synthesis of qualitative studies - BMC Psychiatry." BMC Psychiatry, 28 February 2023, https://bmcpsychiatry.biomedcentral.com/articles/10.1186/s12888-023-04532-2. Accessed 27 February 2025.

"Keeping active." Better Health Channel, https://www.betterhealth.vic.gov.au/healthyliving/keeping-active. Accessed 27 February 2025.

Kim, Eric, et al. "Purpose in life and use of preventive health care services." PNAS, 2014, https://www.pnas.org/content/111/46/16331.full.

Kirkpatrick, Ciera, and Sungkyoung Lee. "Comparisons to picture-perfect motherhood: How Instagram's idealized portrayals of motherhood affect new mothers' well-being." ScienceDirect, vol. 137, 2022, https://www.sciencedirect.com/science/article/abs/pii/S0747563222002394.

Kline, Christopher E. The bidirectional relationship between exercise and sleep: Implications for exercise adherence and sleep improvement, https://pmc.ncbi.nlm.nih.gov/articles/PMC4341978/. Accessed 27 February 2025.

Kuhrt, Matt. "Mental health conditions increase complications and costs of pregnancies, study finds." Fierce Healthcare, 2021, https://www.fiercehealthcare.com/hospitals/mental-health-conditions-increase-complications-and-costs-pregnancies#:~:text=A%20new%20study%20published,complications%20for%20the%20mother%2C.

Lacey, Rebecca, et al. "Social isolation in childhood and adult inflammation: evidence from the National Child Development Study." NIH, 2014, https://pubmed.ncbi.nlm.nih.gov/25197797/.

Leake, Lindsey, et al. "Americans spend 18 years of their adult lives online, according to a new report." Fortune, 6 March 2024, https://fortune.com/well/article/screen-time-over-lifespan/. Accessed 27 February 2025.

Lee, Katherine, et al. "'Lonely within the mother': An exploratory study of first-time mothers' experiences of loneliness." Sage Journals, 2017, https://journals.sagepub.com/doi/abs/10.1177/1359105317723451.

Lemley, Brad. "Interview With Harvard Clinician John Abramson." Discover Magazine, 11 November 2019, https://www.discovermagazine.com/health/interview-with-harvard-clinician-john-abramson. Accessed 27 February 2025.

"List of largest pharmaceutical settlements." Wikipedia, https://en.m.wikipedia.org/wiki/List_of_largest_pharmaceutical_settlements. Accessed 27 February 2025.

"Lung cancer." Better Health Channel, https://www.betterhealth.vic.gov.au/health/conditionsandtreatments/lung-cancer. Accessed 27 February 2025.

"Making one change — getting more fiber — can help with weight loss." Harvard Health, 17 February 2015, https://www.health.harvard.edu/blog/making-one-change-getting-fiber-can-help-weight-loss-201502177721. Accessed 27 February 2025.

Malgorzata Witkowska-Zimny, Malgorzata, et al. "Maternal Sleeping Problems Before and After Childbirth - A Systematic Review." NIH, 2024, https://www.ncbi.nlm.nih.gov/pmc/articles/PMC10918694/.

Martell, Janelle. "Caffeine: How Much is Too Much?" HelpGuide.org, 2024, https://www.helpguide.org/mental-health/wellbeing/how-much-caffeine.

Martin, Joyce A., et al. "National Vital Statistics Reports, Vol. 61, No. 1 (8/2012)." CDC stacks, 28 August 2012, http://www.cdc.gov/nchs/data/nvsr/nvsr61/nvsr61_01.pdf. Accessed 27 February 2025.

McKinlay, John B. "EFFECTS OF PATIENT MEDICATION REQUESTS ON PHYSICIAN PRESCRIBING BEHAVIOR: RESULTS OF A FACTORIAL EXPERIMENT." PubMed Central, 2015, https://www.ncbi.nlm.nih.gov/pmc/articles/PMC4151257/. Accessed 27 February 2025.

Medical News Today. "How sleep deprivation may temporarily ease depression in some people." Medical News Today, 2023, https://www.medicalnewstoday.com/articles/how-sleep-deprivation-may-temporarily-ease-depression-in-some-people#:~:text=%2D%20The%20research%20revealed,the%20brain%2C%20resulting%20in.

"Metabolic syndrome." Better Health Channel, https://www.betterhealth.vic.gov.au/health/conditionsandtreatments/metabolic-syndrome. Accessed 27 February 2025.

Miller, Zach, and Jocelyn Riden. "The Economic Impact of Mental Health on Society." Orlando Treatment Solutions, 10 October 2023, https://orlandotreatmentsolutions.com/the-economic-impact-of-mental-health-on-society/? Accessed 27 February 2025.

"Modest Increases in Kids' Physical Activity Could Avert Billions in Medical and Other Costs." Johns Hopkins, 2017, https://publichealth.jhu.edu/2017/modest-increases-in-kids-physical-activity-could-avert-billions-in-medical-and-other-costs.

MORIN, AMY. "Science Says Finding Your Purpose Could Be the Key to Financial Success." Inc. Magazine, 28 March 2017, https://www.inc.com/amy-morin/you-dont-have-to-choose-between-becoming-wealth-and-doing-something-meaningful-.html. Accessed 27 February 2025.

"Motherly's 2024 State of Motherhood Report." Motherly, 2024, https://www.mother.ly/news/2024-state-of-motherhood-report/.

Mushtaq, Raheel, et al. "Relationship Between Loneliness, Psychiatric Disorders and Physical Health ? A Review on the Psychological Aspects of Loneliness." NIH, 2014, https://www.ncbi.nlm.nih.gov/pmc/articles/PMC4225959/.

Myers, Iris. "EWG's Dirty Dozen Guide to Food Chemicals: The top 12 to avoid." Environmental Working Group, 19 September 2024, https://www.ewg.org/consumer-guides/ewgs-dirty-dozen-guide-food-chemicals-top-12-avoid. Accessed 27 February 2025.

"Overcoming Alcohol Addiction." HelpGuide.org, 5 February 2024, https://www.helpguide.org/mental-health/addiction/overcoming-alcohol-addiction. Accessed 27 February 2025.

Pappas, Stephanie. "The toll of job loss." American Psychological Association, 1 October 2020, https://www.apa.org/monitor/2020/10/toll-job-loss? Accessed 27 February 2025.

Pearson, Rebecca, et al. "Prevalence of Prenatal Depression Symptoms Among 2 Generations of Pregnant Mothers." JAMA Network, https://jamanetwork.com/journals/jamanetworkopen/fullarticle/2687389.

"Perinatal Depression - StatPearls." NCBI, https://www.ncbi.nlm.nih.gov/books/NBK519070/. Accessed 27 February 2025.

Petersen, Andrea. "Why So Many Women in Middle Age Are on Antidepressants." WSJ, 2 April 2022, https://www.wsj.com/articles/why-so-many-middle-aged-women-are-on-antidepressants-11648906393. Accessed 27 February 2025.

"Physical activity." World Health Organization (WHO), 26 June 2024, https://www.who.int/news-room/fact-sheets/detail/physical-activity. Accessed 27 February 2025.

"Physical Activity Guidelines for Americans, 2nd edition." Office of Disease Prevention and Health Promotion, https://health.gov/sites/default/files/2019-09/Physical_Activity_Guidelines_2nd_edition.pdf. Accessed 27 February 2025.

"Plastic Surgery Statistics In USA | Plastic Surgery Facts." Sandeen and Lee Plastic Surgery, https://sandeenandlee.com/blog/plastic-surgery-statistics/. Accessed 27 February 2025.

"Postpartum Period." ScienceDirect, 2014, https://www.sciencedirect.com/topics/agricultural-and-biological-sciences/postpartum-period#:~:text=An%20abrupt%20drop%20in,the%20postpartum%20woman%27s%20poor.

Pratt, Elizabeth, and Daniel Murrell. "Sleep and Immune System." Healthline, 21 February 2019, https://www.healthline.com/health-news/how-sleep-bolsters-your-immune-system. Accessed 27 February 2025.

"Premenstrual Dysphoric Disorder: PMDD Symptoms & Self-Care." HelpGuide.org, 16 January 2025, https://www.helpguide.org/mental-health/depression/premenstrual-dysphoric-disorder-pmdd. Accessed 27 February 2025.

"Refined Carbs and Sugar: Choosing Healthier Carbohydrates." HelpGuide org, 16 January 2025, https://www.helpguide.org/wellness/nutrition/choosing-healthy-carbs. Accessed 27 February 2025.

Reid, Sheldon. "Caffeine and Its Effects on Teenagers." HelpGuide.org, 2024, https://www.helpguide.org/family/parenting/caffeine-and-its-effects-on-teenagers.

"The relationship between sleep and weight loss." Levels Health, 10 June 2022, https://www.levels.com/blog/the-relationship-between-sleep-and-weight-loss. Accessed 27 February 2025.

Sanchez-Vallegas, A., et al. "Physical activity, sedentary index, and mental disorders in the SUN cohort study." Semantic Scholar, 2008, https://pdfs.semanticscholar.org/b086/9f0e2b071fe8063a180edcbd2decec7bdbae.pdf.

Sansone, Randy, and Lori Sansone. "Cosmetic Surgery and Psychological Issues." PMC, 2007, https://pmc.ncbi.nlm.nih.gov/articles/PMC2861519/.

Sardone, Katie. "Katie Sardone, PhD, PMH-C — Behavioral Health Dallas." Behavioral Health Dallas, https://behavioralhealthdallas.com/dr-katie-sardone-psychologist-therapist. Accessed 27 February 2025.

"Sedentary behavior associated with reduced medial temporal lobe thickness in middle-aged and older adults." PLOS, https://journals.plos.org/plosone/article?id=10.1371/journal.pone.0195549#pone.0195549.ref015. Accessed 27 February 2025.

"Sedentary Behavior Research Network (SBRN) – Terminology Consensus Project process and outcome - International Journal of Behavioral Nutrition and Physical Activity." International Journal of Behavioral Nutrition and Physical Activity, 10 June 2017, https://ijbnpa.biomedcentral.com/articles/10.1186/s12966-017-0525-8. Accessed 27 February 2025.

"Sleep for cognitive enhancement." Frontiers, https://www.frontiersin.org/journals/systems-neuroscience/articles/10.3389/fnsys.2014.00046/full. Accessed 27 February 2025.

"Social isolation, loneliness can damage heart and brain health, report says." American Heart Association, 4 August 2022, https://www.heart.org/en/news/2022/08/04/social-isolation-loneliness-can-damage-heart-and-brain-health-report-says. Accessed 27 February 2025.

Spurlock, Morgan, director. Super SIze Me. https://www.youtube.com/watch?v=mlWzDV_0hnU.

"The Startling Statistics." Documenting Hope, https://epidemicanswers.org/about-the-epidemic/the-startling-statistics/. Accessed 27 February 2025.

"Stay Active During Pregnancy: Quick Tips - MyHealthfinder | odphp.health.gov." Office of Disease Prevention and Health Promotion, 1 December 2023, https://odphp.health.gov/myhealthfinder/pregnancy/nutrition-and-physical-activity/stay-active-during-pregnancy-quick-tips. Accessed 27 February 2025.

Steele, Regina. The Mental Mom, http://www.thementalmom.com.

Steptoe, Andrew, and Daisy Fancourt. "Leading a meaningful life at older ages and its relationship with social engagement, prosperity, health, biology, and time use." 2019, https://www.pnas.org/content/116/4/1207.short.

Stotler, Derek, et al. "A Mother's Leadership Legacy: Examining the Mother-To-Child Crossover of Leadership." Georgia State University, 2024, https://news.gsu.edu/2024/05/08/the-leadership-legacy-moms-leave-their-children/#:~:text=Two%20key%20mechanisms%20emerged%20as,confidence%2C%20crucial%20for%20leadership%20success.

Taft, Tiffany. "Depression: Causes, symptoms, treatment, and more." MedicalNewsToday, https://www.medicalnewstoday.com/kc/depression-causes-symptoms-treatments-8933. Accessed 27 February 2025.

"U.S. Overdose Deaths Decrease in 2023, First Time Since 2018." CDC, 15 May 2024, https://www.cdc.gov/nchs/pressroom/nchs_press_releases/2024/20240515.htm. Accessed 27 February 2025.

Valencia, Anna M. "5 Ways Sleep Deprivation Impacts Mental Health in New Mothers." Omega Pediatrics, 2024, https://www.omegapediatrics.com/sleep-deprivation-impact-moms-mentalhealth/#:~:text=Adequate%20sleep%20helps%20the,and%20plays%20a%20role.

"Varicose veins and spider veins." Better Health Channel, https://www.betterhealth.vic.gov.au/health/conditionsandtreatments/varicose-veins-and-spider-veins. Accessed 27 February 2025.

Verhoef, M. J., and E. J. Love. "Women's exercise participation: the relevance of social roles compared to non-role-related determinants." 1992, https://pubmed.ncbi.nlm.nih.gov/1473065/.

Wade, Danielle. "6 Benefits of Stress Management." Psych Central, 25 July 2022, https://psychcentral.com/stress/the-benefits-of-stress-management. Accessed 27 February 2025.

Wade, Danielle. "6 Benefits of Stress Management." Psych Central, 25 July 2022, https://psychcentral.com/stress/the-benefits-of-stress-management. Accessed 27 February 2025.

Wade, Danielle. "6 Benefits of Stress Management." Psych Central, 25 July 2022, https://psychcentral.com/stress/the-benefits-of-stress-management. Accessed 27 February 2025.

Wade, Danielle. "6 Benefits of Stress Management." Psych Central, 25 July 2022, https://psychcentral.com/stress/the-benefits-of-stress-management. Accessed 27 February 2025.

"What is Functional Medicine?" Cleveland Clinic, https://my.clevelandclinic. org/departments/functional-medicine/about. Accessed 27 February 2025.

"When the Bough Breaks: A systematic review and meta-analysis of mental health symptoms in mothers of young children during the COVID-19 pandemic." PubMed Central, https://www.ncbi.nlm.nih.gov/pmc/articles/ PMC9015533/. Accessed 27 February 2025.

"WHO highlights high cost of physical inactivity in first-ever global report.' World Health Organization (WHO), 19 October 2022, https://www.who.int/ news/item/19-10-2022-who-highlights-high-cost-of-physical-inactivity-in-first-ever-global-report? Accessed 27 February 2025.

"Why sleep matters — the economic costs of insufficient sleep: A cross-country comparative analysis." RAND, 30 November 2016, https://www.rand.org/pubs/ research_reports/RR1791.html. Accessed 27 February 2025.

Wilson, Anna, et al. "Baseline Characteristics of a Dyadic Cohort of Mothers With Chronic Pain and Their Children." Clinical Journal of Pain, 2020, https:// journals.lww.com/clinicalpain/abstract/2020/10000/baseline_characteristics_ of_a_dyadic_cohort_of.7.aspx.

Witters, Dan, and SANGEETA AGRAWAL. "Poor Sleep Linked to $44 Billion in Lost Productivity." Gallup, 2022, https://news.gallup.com/ poll/390797/poor-sleep-linked-billion-lost-productivity.aspx?

Wogan, JB. "The Costs of Untreated Maternal Mental Health Conditions." Mathematica, 4 May 2022, https://www.mathematica.org/blogs/the-costs-of-untreated-maternal-mental-health-conditions. Accessed 27 February 2025.

Zhai, Long, et al. "Sedentary behaviour and the risk of depression: a meta-analysis." British Journal of Sports Medicine, 2015, https://bjsm.bmj.com/ content/49/11/705.

www.ingramcontent.com/pod-product-compliance
Lightning Source LLC
Chambersburg PA
CBHW051506120626
46551CB00012B/796